Disclaimer

Before you dive into The Protocol and this book, let's get the legal aspect out of the way. I am not a doctor or medical professional. This book is the sole opinion of the writer and you may or may not obtain the same results. You also may not obtain favorable results. Check with your doctor or doctors, and medical team before proceeding with any or all advice in this book. By continuing and reading this book you assume all liability and waive liability against the author and, or publisher or publishers.

Preface

This book will take you on an incredible journey from knocking on death's door with stage IV cancer to one of triumph as a testament to the power of the human spirit and belief. The metastasis was extensive - brain, lungs, thoracic spine, pancreas, kidneys, adrenal glands, pelvic bone and lymph nodes. Today the tumors have disappeared, shrunk or growth arrested and more importantly - no new metastases in the last year!

Believe me, the healing journey involved hard work, determination and setbacks; however, the one constant was looking for a way where none seemed possible. Today my life is better, but I assure you it is not without challenges. I will forever be grateful to those that came before me and showed me that healing is possible, especially by using food as medicine with natural therapies. Through extensive reading, research and trial and error on myself – The Protocol was born! By combining modern targeted therapies with "The Protocol" I can live my life today and share my story of survival against incredible odds. I will be forever grateful to those that walked with me on this healing journey; and want to share my story and protocol so you can live a healthier fulfilled life.

Acknowledgements

This book is dedicated to those traveling the road to better health and especially those that are battling this horrible life-threatening disease – CANCER!

Believe me when I say I feel blessed and extremely fortunate to be able to write this book, especially given my diagnosis – stage IV cancer with extensive metastasis. During my healing journey it was a whirlwind of turbulent emotions especially during my trips, office visits, diagnostic scans and lab work. At times I felt alone and that no one truly understood what I was experiencing physically, and especially emotionally.

Despite this, I was very fortunate to have family, friends and previous coworkers in my corner that gave me unwavering support and lifted my spirits when I needed it the most!

Starting with my incredible mother who is a true God send and never left my side especially when I was bedridden. Completely supporting me in my new lifestyle changes, especially by making me my keto plant-based meals without question! Words cannot describe the gratitude, appreciation and love I have for her!

To my sister and her family, The Gemoets who gave continual support and traveled with me to the Gerson based clinic in Baja Tijuana Mexico – Thank you - you guys are Awesomeness! A huge thank you to CHIPSA who started me on the right path with organic plant-based foods and IV Vitamin C. This became an integral part of my healing journey. Of course, I adjusted and augmented based

3

on scan results and the rest is fortunately a living testament to the body's innate healing capacity when nourished with the appropriate foods!

To my cousin Rose Elena C and Irma A. who helped me on my travel and stay in Mexico and have continuously supported me – con todo corazon, muchas gracias!

I would be completely remiss if I did not acknowledge my close and dear friends who were there for me every step of the way. My cousin Jose G. who countless times unselfishly took me to my Dr. appointments for support and because I was unable to drive myself. To my brother from another mother Fonso T. who called me daily to see how I was doing and drove to San Diego to support me on my trips to CHIPSA in Baja Tijuana Mx. To Gary K. who called me daily to check on me and see if I needed anything – his continued support is truly appreciated. To my brother Jorge who takes time to check in on me – Thank You hermano!

To Wissam E. for all the conversations and calls to help me navigate the emotional turmoil, life changes and give me new perspective - much love and appreciation amigo!

I also appreciate those that routinely took time to visit with me or call routinely to say hi; thank you Donnell W, Maria G, Maria M, Marisol C, Margarita V, Claudia V, Abel G, Phil G, Joe C, Scotty Mac, Martina P, Melissa L, Dave Z, Casey M, Larry P, Carlos C, and Genaro G. To my previous co-workers Marcus, Bernie and Stilly who took up a collection for me at my previous job – Thank you! A special thank you to my union brothers and sisters; the USW 7-1 board members, and especially Eric S, Shawn S and Brain U for their unwavering support.

To Northwestern Memorial Hospital and its practitioners, specifically Dr. Sosman and his team; Dr. Alexis Larson, Dr. Sachdev, and Dr Vikram

Aggarwal - Thank you! The modern targeted therapies, consults, lab work and diagnostics helped treat and guide me!

To Dr. Ali Al Khazaali, a local endocrinologist who assisted in guiding treatments to prevent severe dehydration and thus severe kidney issues or nephrectomy - Thank you!

To the wonderful staff at Float Sixty in northwest indiana where I do my weekly cryotherapy - thank you Kara, Abbie, John, Ricky, Jessica and Issa!

To an incredible person and NP, Stacy Taylor at NWI Integrative Health & Wellness (formally NWI IV Drip Spa) and her staff for providing alternative treatments including my IV Vitamin C which is truly a lifesaver! Please keep doing what you do – the world needs you!

Finally to my kindred spirit, pharmacist Saira Z who helped with editing, research and putting my words and thoughts to paper. Thank you for helping me document my journey and protocol so it can be shared with others in the hopes of helping people live long fruitful lives.

Words can never fully express my gratitude to all of the people that have given their support on my journey! This list is not comprehensive as I was and am fortunate to have friends and acquaintances who check in on me – thank you! It has been a long tumultuous challenging road full of emotions, setbacks and triumphs - the support has been heartfelt!

Thank you all for your kind words and time – especially your time, for it is the one thing that we can never get more of!

With much love and appreciation!

Javier Almendarez
CANCER Survivor and Thriver

Table of Contents

Foreword

This book is dedicated to all who are on the journey to better themselves by becoming a healthier and fit YOU! Whether you want to feel better, look better, or just plain tired of not feeling well, believe in yourself, have faith, and stay on the path. Above all - love yourself and start the journey wherever you are. It is your path alone! After years of going back and forth with fad diets, gimmick exercise routines and workout equipment, I finally got the worst wake-up call – stage IV CANCER. My answer lied in a complete overhaul of my eating and lifestyle and this time it was no quick fix or gimmick - my life literally depended on it!

Javier Almendarez

Introduction

You can be a victim of cancer or you can be a survivor and thriver from cancer -
the choice is yours!

JA

One can either succumb to the clutches of cancer or emerge triumphant as its survivor and thriver. I stand before you today as living proof, a testament to resilience and the indomitable spirit that resides within us all.

However, when I got the diagnosis, I was far from being the person you see now. In fact, I was the complete opposite. Let's rewind to day #1, so you can embark on this journey from the beginning with me.

September 2020: Picture this: a dimly lit hospital room, the air heavy with the weight of an impending storm. I was perched on the edge of a bed, the world crumbling around me. The shadows of fear danced menacingly, whispering these exact words repeatedly:

Cancer- Stage IV.

Aggressive. Incurable. Deadly!

You know that feeling when you are caught in the unrelenting grip of an unyielding nightmare? That was me, right there at that moment. A million thoughts flashed through my mind, but none escaped my lips. Was this my time? Would I just give in, or would I fight? It was a daunting thought, and it took me time to process - I knew I would be in the fight of my life - literally! Who would have thought I, Javier Almendarez, would fall prey to this monster? At least not me. Terror washed over my body in waves, with the world's weight pressing down on me.

Even as the haunting words of my doctor kept echoing in my ears, a nagging thought streaked through my mind. How did this happen? How did I reach this? How did I end up here in this hospital with cancer, of all the diseases and disorders - why me, God?

****

It all Started with a Cheeseburger

Rewind to the events that landed me in the hospital diagnosed with Stage IV cancer. Tired from my midnight shift and heading home exhausted, I suddenly craved one of my favorite meals: cheeseburgers and French fries. I picked up the food and headed home to watch TV before falling asleep and enjoying my long weekend. I ate the food and went to bed, *sounds domestic and boring, right?* This couldn't be further from the truth - my life was about to change forever!

Unfortunately, that would be the last time I would have *a normal* moment for a long time. Shortly after laying down, I felt an odd sensation in my throat, and thinking it was just phlegm, I sprung out of bed to spit it out. Out came phlegm, *so I thought*, but it was phlegm tainted with globs of bright red blood. Bright red blood out of my mouth, sparkling, even evilly winking at me.

"Could be a pimple bursting," I told myself. I needed to get a grip. It happens to the best of us. I went back to bed.

How wrong was I…?

The phlegm and bright red blood just would not stop, and now the alarm bells started ringing for real. It was my moment to freak out, and I did. I called the ambulance; the thought of me drowning in my blood was just too much for me.

However, in five minutes *[yes, I remember the details]*, my spit was back to normal with no blood. Almost as if nothing had happened!

Nevertheless, the bright red blood specks were still dancing in my head, and I decided to proceed with the checkup primarily because of the fear of the recurrence of such an event.

Ambulance arrives. Cursory checks. Vitals are okay. All is good.

I went back to watching TV just to soothe my jittery nerves. However, subconsciously, I had made a decision. I had to go to the ER; this was far from normal!

****

Wishful Thinking is One Thing; Reality Another

Nervousness and uneasiness were my companions on my way to the ER.

After listening to my narration of events at the hospital, blood samples were collected, and chest X-rays were taken to ensure there was nothing wrong on the pulmonary front.

A barrage of conflicting thoughts erupted as I fidgeted in the waiting room.

"Ah, man, there you are, everything is ok, it is just an odd occurrence, we are sure there is nothing wrong with you," One voice whispered in my mind wishfully.

But a more sinister voice whispered in my mind simultaneously, *"How sure are you?"*

You may understand my situation. When experiencing these thoughts, I was in denial about the event's seriousness and tried to push it off as a one-time occurrence.

14

However, the reports and the doctor to interpret these reports soon arrived, and the inevitable truth was out.

As I would find several full body scans later, I had the c-word disease - Cancer!

Not just cancer but stage IV kidney cancer that had spread to my brain, lungs, pancreas, hip bone, thoracic spine, kidneys, adrenal glands and lymph nodes.

****

Face Reality as it is, Not as it was or as You Wish it to be

Grief, despair, and similar synonyms became meaningless to me that day. They could not describe what I was feeling.

My world was shattered!

World. Earth. The amazing people that walk on this earth. Friends, family, colleagues. People with whom I talked, laughed, and enjoyed a cheeseburger. Everything was going to disappear in no time.

Cheeseburger, *there was something funny there*. It sparked in my brain shortly, but the grief was too overwhelming for any sane thought to prevail.

Tears welled in my eyes; even if I had tried restraint, it would not have worked. Each falling drop was a testament to the tumultuous storm whirling within me. I was not the glass half-empty type, but at that time, life's unfairness screamed in my life the loudest.

****

It's not a Posthumous Account of my Sufferings, by the way!

And if your bewilderment is borderline with doubts over my sanity, I completely understand. After all, I had cancer spread all over my body. I should not have lasted a year, let alone over three and one-half years!.

15

Well, here is how I made mournful shadows of gloom my friends that awful night.

I could be a cancer victim, or I could be a cancer survivor and thriver. It all depended on my mental strength and perspective. Now was a very good time to prove my mettle. As Christopher Reeve says,

"Once you choose hope, anything is possible."

The aura around me resonated with my newfound determination when I started thinking on these lines. Darkness dispelled, even if a little bit and a glimmer of hope broke through the darkness.

And that was all I needed.

Knowing is Not Enough - You Must Take Action

Mahatma Gandhi said, "Your future depends on what you do today."

So, it was going to be a long journey and not one that could be accomplished using the usual elements in the toolkit for cancer survival. No, they were not working for people around me; it had to be something else.

Let me tell you, my story is of a scared man who turned his darkest hour into a testament of strength, resilience, and hope. It was not easy; I relied on trials and tests, probably more than any hospital would have typically done.

I invite you to embark on this journey with me as I unveil the chapters of my life where I defied the odds, discovered the power of nourishing both body and soul, and got another crack at life.

Oh, and remember one thing*: cheeseburgers are very important in our story!*

Chapter 1: A Life Shattered

The introduction may seem like a solitary chapter only. But for me, it was the beginning of a new life where there wasn't much normal.

Stage IV cancer. The more I tried not to think about it, the more these words started to dance in front of me like a death sentence. It was as if denial washed over me like a tidal wave. I will admit that I haven't been diligent about my health, but it wasn't as if I completely ignored it. I visited my primary physician regularly and even had yearly physicals at my workplace.

Could the diagnosis be a mistake, though? At any cost, I had to get a second opinion.

Denial is not a River in Egypt

My family has a history of tuberous sclerosis. To avoid the medical jargon, we can say that it is a condition that leads to non-cancerous tumors. I clung to this glimmer of hope as well. I desperately prayed that this condition might shield me from the darkness looming over my life.

However, what happened in the following days shattered my fragile illusion of normalcy, to say the very least. It was as if the harsh reality of my diagnosis began to sink in slowly. A biopsy was taken, and the results were proven to be conclusive. It extinguished every sliver of hope I had.

Truth, after all, cannot be escaped from, I learned.

****

Probing the Extent of Damage

The worst thing about a cancer diagnosis is that things only worsen after the diagnosis. Now, it was game time for my oncologists, who ordered a battery of tests. The idea was to gauge the extent of the cancer's reach within my body. As I mentioned earlier, the results of these tests were chilling. The cancer had metastasized to my brain, lungs, pancreas, bone, kidneys, thoracic spine, adrenal glands and lymph nodes.

Someone had taken my breath away, it seemed. A dark cloud with its ominous shadows had spread over my life, over every corner of my body.

Could I ever get out of this trap, this relentless storm? I had no shelter in sight.

****

Cancer is Confusing

The following weeks were filled with countless hours of internet research and consultations with medical professionals. As I would understand and realize later, cancer was slowly becoming my obsession. I wanted to understand how I fell prey to this terrible condition. From the night I coughed up bloody phlegm to lying under an MRI machine, I had traveled a lot, even though only a few weeks had passed.

Here, I would like to pause upon my gloomy reflections and share something about the silent killer that renal cancer is. Renal or kidney cancer is like a hidden monster; it lurks undetected in the body, showing little indication of its presence. Then, one day, suddenly, it infiltrates other vital organs, and symptoms appear. It is only then you realize the monster that laid dormant! But here is the thing about symptoms, even if other common health concerns mask them. Like in my case, it was bloody phlegm that I thought was a burst pimple. Oh, and did I mention my exhaustive feelings? I always thought it was because of the work. But well, the revelations were enough to solidify the severity of my situation.

18

The American Cancer Society says about renal cancer in 2023:

https://www.cancer.org/cancer/types/kidney-cancer/about/key-statistics.html

"About 81,800 new cases of kidney cancer (52,360 in men and 29,440 in women) will be diagnosed. About 14,890 people (9,920 men and 4,970 women) will die from this disease.

These numbers include all types of kidney and renal pelvis cancers. Most people with kidney cancer are older. The average age of people when diagnosed is 64, with most people being diagnosed between ages 65 and 74. Kidney cancer is very uncommon in people younger than age 45. Kidney cancer is about twice as common in men as in women and more common in African Americans, American Indians, and Alaska Natives."

****

I Felt Every Emotion in the World - from Despair to Hope, from Anger to Happiness

Today, I stare at a sky littered with stars as I write these words. It fills me with absolute joy.

But a few years ago, I stared at a similar sky, and my heart was drenched with misery and grief.

Now that I think about that time, I was at a crossroads. I had a decision to make and soon. Succumb to the despair or find the strength to fight back? Of course, I had to fight back. But finding the strength to fight back was the main issue. I was experiencing a full spectrum of emotions, from anger to helplessness, hope to depression.

And then, one day, I realized something. I had to let these feelings wash over me. They were an integral part of my journey. And once wallowing in self-pity was done, I had to get up and get going. Grief and despair would not solve the problem, and the problem here was such that my life depended on it. In common problems, we have the luxury of time; this was different. I needed to make a decision soon, and I did it.

****

The Clock was Ticking Mercilessly

The first step that I took was to visit a local oncologist. I was determined not to waste time, my precious time, in carelessness like a pulmonologist did previously by performing improper and inconclusive biopsies on my lung. Previous studies had indicated the cancer started in my kidneys and that is where the biopsy should have been initially performed!

However, the first experience was not that amazing. Now that I think back, the oncologist seemed more interested in starting my treatment rather than explaining the deadly disease to me in detail. The first step the oncologist suggested was to implant a port for chemotherapy. But, I had read enough and seen enough patients undergoing chemotherapy to understand that this would not solve my problem. It will limit my movement and make me a person who is constantly reminded of their condition physically. Through my reading and research, I also realized that movement was critical to healing. I did not want anything that would impede movement or be a constant reminder of the battle I was facing demoralizing me - it was a challenging enough situation without an ever-present reminder. So, after careful consideration, I sought options that worked synergistically with my body.

Fortunately for me, I live near Chicago. I have access to nationally recognized hospitals equipped with cutting-edge medical science techniques. I had a recommendation, and through this recommendation, I found a treatment plan that aligned with my goals. It would be in IV infusion that would not require a port and be performed monthly.

Killing Cancer - One Cocktail at a Time

My treatment plan consisted of an immunotherapy cocktail of Opdivo and Yervoy. It was administered once every four weeks. The first treatment went well, and thankfully, no port was needed!

Opdivo and Yervoy, the dynamic immunotherapeutic duo, assumed pivotal roles in my relentless battle against cancer. Opdivo, a potent checkpoint inhibitor, wielded the power to rekindle my immune system's vigilance by neutralizing the immune checkpoints exploited by cancer cells. Each infusion of this medication introduced a cautious yet hopeful perspective, marking a potential turning point in my treatment. Opdivo's side effects remained relatively mild, affording me precious moments of normalcy amid the pervasive uncertainty(Kahl, 2020).

Yervoy, a collaborator in this scientific endeavor, complemented Opdivo's actions by targeting distinct immune checkpoints, amplifying the immune system's response against malignant cells. The calculated synergy of these two medications was challenging, including pronounced side effects that precipitated overwhelming fatigue and a questioning of the chosen path ("Ipilimumab (Yervoy) in Combination with Nivolumab (Opdivo) for the First-Line Treatment of Advanced Renal Cell Cancer," 2019).

Probably the first time I felt a little cheery and full of hope was during this treatment when I realized that the therapy did not have any side effects initially, and I felt the same for a couple of months. I finally thought I would get this deadly disease under control at the least and prayed I would be rid of it once and for all!

Making Critical Decisions Echoing with My Inner Peace

They say good decisions come from experience and experience comes from bad decisions, which was true in my case.

I was optimistic and anxiously awaited the next scan due in approximately three months.

However, there was no good news. I developed a strong reaction after my second infusion treatment, but I knew there would be some cost, at the very least.

The side effects I experienced included extreme exhaustion and unusually strong shivers.

The shivers were to the point that I felt I might need to go to the ER. Fortunately, they subsided but left me lethargic to the point where I had to take a leave of absence.

Work was missing from life now. One vital element of my life was already gone.

I could no longer work properly or even drive. However, things were not extremely bad. I could still do the basic chores of life and engage in activities such as eating or bathing on my own, but it was becoming more and more complex with each day passing.

The doctor and I decided to skip a monthly round of the regiment due to the side effects, which was fine with me. After the fourth treatment, the regimen went to only the Opdivo on a 30-day intravenous basis with no port required. I started treatment in early November 2020 but the scans did not show the regression that the doctor or I hoped for, and now I had to decide to stay the course for a while longer or choose alternative treatments I had read about earlier.

Things were not horrible, but they were not what I had hoped for. It was a while before we could be sure of anything. But I had done something incredible already; I refused traditional chemo and decided to take an alternative route. Only time was going to tell if that was a wise option or not.

Chapter 2: A Ride to Mexico

Putting Paradigm Shifts in Perspective

As the conventional cancer treatment continued, fear gripped my whole being. I had a strong hunch that this path would not lead me to the outcomes I was desperately waiting for.

I had numerous consultations with multiple oncologists, and all pointed to the same pharmacological treatment - which, in my case, was not showing tumor regression. Then, I decided to put my money into holistic alternative treatment.

A three-week outpatient treatment abroad, *let us give it a go, I thought.*

This treatment center was rooted in the Gerson protocol but incorporated additional therapies as medical knowledge advanced. However, the core idea remained rooted in empowering the body to heal itself. In addition, they said I could continue my immunotherapy.

The mantra at that particular moment in my treatment was - my body has an innate ability to help heal itself - USE IT!

A Ride to Mexico

Was it easy, you ask?

Not at all.

The decision to seek alternative treatments in Mexico was probably the toughest one I have taken in my entire life. As you can imagine, my body was a battlefield; the onslaught of cancer practically destroyed my body. Waking up every day was proving to be a gruelling challenge, let alone thinking about the foreign healthcare landscape south of the border.

However, there was some hope, a promise of a different approach to healing that encouraged me to embark on a journey that would hopefully reclaim my health.

Reaching the Coast of Hope

The journey cost me quite a bit, financially and physically. My American insurance did not cover the unconventional treatment I had opted for, so I had to cough up over $30,000 - US dollars - not pesos mind you!

Quite a substantial sum, but I felt I had no choice and needed to do it!

The cancer treatments that I had undergone in the United States were far from effective. I wanted something more practical. I had a few consultations with Mexican doctors, which gave me a glimmer of optimism. It appeared as if their approach, combined with the immunotherapy treatment I was receiving in the U.S., might accelerate my recovery.

Then there was the journey itself. It tested my strength like nothing else. Now, I was physically weakened, and my memory had started to play tricks on me, but I knew that things would not work out well for me if I did not keep moving forward.

Sometimes, You Have to Take a Leap of Faith

It was not entirely unknown to me, though.

All my life, I had been aware of alternative treatments that veered from the conventional paths, such as chemotherapy and radiation. Now, these holistic therapies always appeared to me as kinder alternatives.

However, the cost associated with them was significantly higher because they were not available at home but abroad and also not covered by my health insurance. Hence, before investing a substantial amount of money, I should explore the latest conventional treatment, i.e., immunotherapy. Immunotherapy gave better results than traditional chemotherapy, and from the preliminary research I had conducted on my own, immunotherapy was a more sustainable path to healing(Sordo-Bahamonde et al., 2023). Additionally, immunotherapy was in line with my philosophy of helping my body help itself heal and do no or minimal harm to my body.

The Power of Knowledge

For once, Cersei Lannister was not correct.

Knowledge IS power.

I spent most of my time trying to learn all about cancer types, treatments, and the role of nutrition in cancer treatment. To me, the importance of informed decisions was more evident than ever. Navigating the complex landscape of modern medicine and alternative treatments to counter this many-headed monster is only possible by reading a lot. And that is what I did, too!

Medical research tells us that when it comes to cancer, the crux of the matter is hidden in how our immune system corresponds to each treatment(Liu & Zeng, 2012).

Take chemotherapy, for example, which is effective in some cases but can compromise the immune system. It has a crippling effect on your immune system, leaving it less equipped to defend against the possibility of cancer returning(Wargo et al., 2015).

To be completely honest with you, this thought troubled me the most. From personal experience, I have known many folks undergoing chemotherapy who only suffered from a relapse or succumbed to the disease.

Now that I knew this, it was time to start an immunotherapy trial. I knew that for the sake of my health, I had to try these new options, even though the associated costs were monumental.

Only One Who Makes Quick Decisions Survives

So many moons passed, but the cancer showed no signs of relenting. For me, this was a signal that I must consider an alternative path. I was willing to adapt and embrace any new approaches that could help me survive.

Yet, I must repeat it: my decisions were not taken lightly.

My life was uncertain. What an odd way of putting things in perspective….

However, I needed clarification on what I was doing.

I cannot help but remember the moments when I had to set aside my old ways of thinking to do what was best for me. Making these choices also meant considering the perspectives of those providing advice. Modern medicine often leans on pharmaceuticals as the primary treatment modality. In contrast, alternative medicine takes a holistic, whole-body approach, putting faith in the body's ability to heal under the right conditions and with proper nutrition. The body possesses an innate, built-in self-healing program, ready to guide us through life's challenges. I had adopted my philosophy moving forward: "Use my body's innate ability to heal itself and to treat the body the way it was designed to be treated"! [More on this later]

The Concept of Food

I think now is the perfect time to discuss food's importance.

Well, it is always essential, but at this point, it is even more so because we are talking about a deadly disease that is now thought to be shaped by what we eat.

The diet that we eat today is mainly processed unnatural foods, especially in the US.

Would you agree if I tell you that it has instead led us astray from what our bodies were designed to consume in the first place?

Ask yourself this question.

"Was my body designed to eat this?"

I believe you know the answer already.

This question distinguishes our contemporary diet from what our bodies have evolved to ingest.

Do you think our ancestors had metabolic systems capable of processing highly refined, nutrient-poor foods such as burgers, sweetened carbonated drinks, pizzas, etc?

No, they were not.

Food Stories, But of Different Kinds

There was no hiding from the fact that I eventually had to embark on a transformation in my dietary habits.

For those who are suffering from cancer, there is one point that I would love to speak about repeatedly—nutrition matters.

Here, I am not referring to the standard American diet we usually eat when I speak of nutrition. Instead, it is about going the opposite way. It is about asking this question repeatedly.

Was my body designed to eat this? Is your body designed to adapt to any of that cheeseburger you had for lunch, that ice cream you had at night, that sugar-loaded coffee you drank early in the morning?

And my dear, if the answers that you are getting are negative, well, you must start your transformation right away.

This dietary transformation will hopefully unveil a profound lesson for you—food matters.

For me, I learned it the hard way, the value of nutritious eating. It was during my alternative treatment that my eyes were finally fully opened. And once you start learning, you continue to learn and have "aha" moments daily because of the invaluable lessons in the "food as medicine" niche, as I did during my alternative therapy(Downer et al., 2020).

During my journey, I had the opportunity to have a genetic test of my tumor biopsy. It revealed that my cancer type primarily used sugar as fuel. This finding resonated with my research on intermittent fasting as a health-promoting practice. I realized it was not just good but excellent for me, as it lowered my blood glucose levels, cutting off the primary food source for my cancer type.

Unlocking the Benefits of Intermittent Fasting

Intermittent fasting became a pivotal aspect of my daily routine. I typically followed a 16-hour fast with an 8-hour eating window, usually consisting of only one or two small meals.   Sometimes, I extended the fast to 20 hours without feeling hungry or fatigued.

Understanding that I did not abruptly transition to this fasting schedule is crucial(Welton et al., 2020).

I started by ceasing eating at 7 p.m. and delaying my breakfast until after 8 a.m. the next day, gradually extending the fasting window each week. Currently, I fast daily from 8 p.m. until 1 p.m. or later the next day. Currently, I fast two days a week and administer IV Vitamin C after a 16hr fast and continue fasting for the remainder of the 48hrs .

One notable difference I experienced after adopting an authentic, natural, and unprocessed food diet was the waning of food cravings. I no longer desired or craved processed foods as I once did. Despite my love for pizza, I did not yearn for it or other processed foods. It was a transformation driven by the power of conscious dietary choices.

29

The Fundamental Truth

In my narrative, food remains a central theme, underlining its pivotal role in a healthy body and life. The age-old adage that "you are what you eat" has never been more relevant, especially in the context of health. Today, as we grapple with the complexities of health and disease, the understanding that "food is medicine" has never been more profound. It's a truth we all need to grasp and apply.

A Glimpse of the Future

My battle against cancer is an intersection of traditional and alternative treatments, the transformative power of nutrition, and my unwavering determination created a tapestry of experiences and insights.

Together, these elements formed the foundation of my journey toward recovery.

The road ahead was riddled with challenges, but my spirit was rekindling.

In the following lines, I want to describe all the dimensions of my battle against cancer. While you will get all the details in the chapters to follow, each chapter will give you a deeper insight into the resilience of the human spirit and the unwavering will to live when confronted with the ultimate threat: death.

Chapter 3: Understanding Cancer

A stage IV cancer diagnosis is a revelation that can shatter your whole world. The diagnosis signifies the advanced and metastatic stage of cancer. It is the point at which the disease has spread beyond the primary tumor stage. Now, it is multiple areas of the body and in my case, pretty much everywhere! The cancer diagnosis at any stage is a tough challenge. But, a stage IV diagnosis is particularly challenging, given the advanced nature of the disease. Before I go on about how I found a way to return to everyday life, it is sensible to discuss stage IV cancer a little bit more and look at some of the causes and treatment options that are currently available. I will also talk about why some of the current treatment options are not the wisest course of action to counter cancer at this stage, in my opinion.

Here's What Happens in Your Body at Cancer Stage IV

Stage IV cancer is mostly about metastasis(Brand, 2019).

Metastasis is the process by which cancer cells break away from the primary tumor. Cancer cells can then enter the bloodstream or the lymphatic system of the human body and travel to the other parts of the body(Welch & Hurst, 2019).

Metastasis is a complex process; it involves various molecular and cellular mechanisms. Because metastatic cancer cells can find home in different organs of the human body, they can form secondary tumors quite quickly. Some factors that could influence the likelihood of metastasis include:

- the type of cancer you're dealing with,
- its diagnosis stage, and
- the patient's overall health.

A significant contributing factor to stage IV cancer is the late diagnosis. A better prognosis for most cancers is possible when they are detected in their early stage. But unfortunately, as it was in my case, cancer was already at an advanced stage. And it had eluded my body's medical attention in the preceding years. So, naturally, the treatment for stage IV cancer is challenging, and the existing treatment is a lot less effective(Brand, 2019).

Some other barriers that might be there when we talk about stage IV cancer diagnosis include:

- Lack of awareness
- Financial constraints
- Fear of medical procedures or conceptions about cancer

In my case, perhaps, the lack of awareness is the most enormous box to check.

This is What You Experience at Stage IV

Let me tell you a little about what I was feeling during stage IV cancer and what you, unfortunately, are likely to see if you have succumbed to this state of cancer.

Pain is, of course, one of the most prevalent symptoms in this stage. Cancer grows, and it spreads to distant sites. And as it spreads, it leads to discomfort. The nature of this discomfort can be both local and general. Usually, the pain results from tumor compression over the years by organs. Nerve compression also happens, releasing inflammatory substances where the cancer cells aggravate pain(Gilbert et al., 1978).

Stage IV cancer often brings severe fatigue as well. As the disease progresses, the stress of treatment can always exhaust a patient. The exhaustion is not just physical but emotional as well. Over time, this fatigue can become a chronic issue and impact your daily life.

You will likely lose weight, but not at an average rate. You'll lose weight at an unprecedented rate, in an unprecedented manner. Your body's metabolic responses also change. Your appetite is reduced significantly, and cancer's energy consumption contributes massively to weight loss. This is quite concerning because good nutrition is crucial for your overall well-being, cancer or no cancer.

Now let us talk about some of the more serious symptoms, primarily of respiratory and gastrointestinal nature. When you are experiencing advanced lung cancer, for example, your respiratory symptoms are more prevalent than other symptoms. Some of these symptoms include shortness of breath and puffing. But, if you feel frequent chest pain and cannot breathe properly, this is a sign that something serious is wrong with you. Lung involvement often severely impacts your quality of life(Koo et al., 2020).

Then, cancers that affect the gastrointestinal tract or metastasize to the digestive system are also responsible for symptoms such as nausea and abdominal pain. Frequent constipation or diarrhea can make it difficult for you to eat and maintain proper nutrition. In my case, I had diarrhea caused by a diuretic in my blood pressure medication! This caused severe dehydration that severely affected my kidney function. Fortunately, an Endocrinologist removed the HTCZ from my medication and the kidney function started to improve.

Sometimes, you're likely to experience neurological symptoms as well. For example, if cancer metastasizes to your brain or spinal cord, you'll likely experience neurological symptoms. Some of these symptoms include headaches, weakness, seizures, or sometimes predominant changes in cognitive function. These symptoms are quite distressing, as you can imagine. They affect your overall ability to carry out daily activities quite severely. Additionally, in my case (renal cancer) memory and fatigue were an issue; this is common due to the nature of treatments (Koo et al., 2020).

This is How Cancer is Diagnosed

Now, for those who are unaware of how cancer diagnosis usually takes place, let me explain how diagnosis at stage IV cancer typically happens. Usually, it will involve a combination of medical history, physical examination, imaging studies, and laboratory tests. Let me talk about the primary diagnostic tools and steps involved in the following lines of this brief.

The first thing to talk about is the imaging studies. These studies are crucial for staging and determining how much the cancer has spread in your body. Some imaging modalities used include computed tomography (CT) scans, magnetic resonance imaging (MRI), positron emission tomography (PET), and bone scans. Typically, ultrasound scans are also used to assess certain cancers as well.

Let us talk about these imaging modalities a little bit more. Computed tomography scans, commonly known as CT scans, provide detailed cross-sectional images of our body. They could help locate tumors and evaluate their sizes.

Then, there is an MRI, a high-resolution imaging technique to assess tumors in our body's soft tissues. By soft tissues, I mean the brain and spinal cord. PET scans are used for highlighting areas with high metabolic activity. These techniques use a radioactive tracer to highlight this high metabolic activity, indicating cancerous growth. Finally, bone scans are used to detect metastasis in cases where cancer has spread in the bones already. I mentioned the ultrasound techniques earlier; they are usually employed to assess certain types of cancers, mainly in the abdomen and pelvis region.

If you have been unfortunate enough to know a family or friend who has cancer, a biopsy is one of the most commonly used words you might have come across. A biopsy is one of the most definitive ways to confirm the presence of cancer. Not only does it confirm the presence of cancer, but it is also helpful in determining the cancer type. While taking the biopsy, a small tissue sample is collected from a tumor or the nearby affected area. This sample is then examined under a microscope. Pathologists usually perform this analysis to identify cancer cells and determine which cancer you suffer from.

Often, blood tests are also conducted to check for markers of cancer. Usually, an elevated level of specific proteins or tumor-specific antigens (TSAs) in blood gives a clue about cancers. These blood tests are helpful in cancer diagnosis and the overall response of the human body to cancer treatment(Medina-Lara et al., 2020).

Staging the Cancer

It is like giving a number to your cancer. Oncologists use Roman numerals from 0 to IV. Stage IV cancer is a cancer that has spread to distant sites in our body. Usually, staging is a process that takes into account many factors. Some of these factors are the size of the primary tumor, the extent of lymph node involvement, and the presence of metastasis.

Insights into Medical Treatment Options Available

1. Chemotherapy

- **How it works**

Chemotherapy relies on powerful drugs to kill or, at least, slow down the growth of cancer cells. These drugs target rapidly dividing cells, which are a hallmark of cancer cells. Chemotherapy can be administered orally or intravenously, circulating throughout the body(Amjad et al., 2023).

- **Types**

Different chemotherapy drugs may be used depending on the specific cancer. Some of the most commonly used chemotherapeutic drugs include:

- ❖ Cisplatin
- ❖ Dyclophosphamide

- ❖ Dacarbazine
- ❖ Ifosfamide
- ❖ Lomustine
- ❖ Melphalan
- ❖ Temozolomide
- ❖ Trabectedin

- **Possible Limitations**

  Treatment Resistance: Cancer cells can develop resistance to treatments over time; this reduces the overall effectiveness of chemotherapy by a great extent. Oncologists must adjust treatment plans in such a scenario, switch to different drugs, or explore new therapeutic options through clinical trials.

  Toxicity: Chemotherapy and radiation therapy can have toxic effects on healthy cells, which affect the patient's quality of life. Supportive care measures and medications can help manage and alleviate side effects, but this often comes at the cost of dose adjustments and treatment breaks, thereby extending the duration of the cancer treatment significantly.

  Limited Effectiveness: In some cases, primarily when the cancer has spread extensively, treatments may provide only limited benefit, and the primary goal may shift from curing the disease to taking care of symptoms. That is something that I did not like about the conventional treatments the most(Marin et al., 2009).

2. Targeted Therapy

- **How it works**

  Targeted therapy relies on the drugs that specifically target the molecular and genetic abnormalities within cancer cells. These drugs interfere with the cellular signaling pathways responsible for cancer growth with minimal impact on normal cells (Shuel, 2022).

- **Types**

Different targeted therapies are developed for specific cancer types. Monoclonal antibodies and small molecule drugs are pretty important in this list.

- **Possible Limitations**

Treatment Resistance: Targeted therapies may face challenges when cancer cells develop resistance over time. Adjusting treatment plans or exploring new therapeutic options through clinical trials then becomes very important.

Side Effects: While targeted therapy tends to have fewer side effects than chemotherapy, it can still lead to immune-related adverse events, skin rashes, hypertension and gastrointestinal issues. Regular monitoring and prompt management of side effects are essential.

3. Immunotherapy

- **How it works**

Immunotherapy harnesses the body's immune system to recognize and attack cancer cells. These include immune checkpoint inhibitors, monoclonal antibodies, and cancer vaccines.

- **Types**

Immunotherapy has been extensively researched recently and is now employed for various cancers.

- **Possible Limitations**

Immune-Related Side Effects: Immunotherapy can trigger immune-related adverse events that affect various organs and systems, leading to conditions like colitis, pneumonitis, or thyroid problems.

Limited Response: Not all patients respond to immunotherapy; some cancers resist these treatments. Ongoing research aims to improve response rates and expand the application of immunotherapies(Curigliano & Criscitiello, 2014).

4. Hormone Therapy

- **How it works**

  Hormone therapy is mainly used for hormone-related cancers like breast and prostate cancer. It involves medications that block or lower the levels of hormones fueling cancer growth("Hormone Replacement Therapy and Cancer," 2001).

- **Types**

  Tamoxifen and aromatase inhibitors are commonly used for breast cancer, androgen deprivation therapy is often used for prostate cancer treatment.

- **Possible Limitations**

  Hormone Resistance: Over time, some cancers may become resistant to hormone therapy, leading to disease progression. Oncologists may explore alternative hormonal treatments or combine different therapies to overcome resistance.

  Side Effects: Hormone therapy can lead to side effects like hot flashes, osteoporosis, and sexual dysfunction("Hormone Replacement Therapy and Cancer," 2001).

5. Radiation Therapy

- **How it works**

  Radiation therapy uses high-energy beams to target and destroy cancer cells. It often alleviates symptoms or shrinks tumors but often leads to the sensations of pain and pressure.

- **Types**

  External beam radiation and brachytherapy are the two key types of radiation therapy.

- **Possible Limitations**

  Localized Treatment: Radiation therapy is a localized treatment, and it may not be effective for cancers that have spread widely throughout the body.

Side Effects: Radiation therapy can cause side effects specific to the treated area, such as skin irritation, fatigue, and localized discomfort(Jaffray & Gospodarowicz, 2015).

6. Palliative Care

- **How it works**

Palliative care focuses on symptom management and improving the quality of life but it does not cure the underlying cancer. It is all about providing comfort and support.

- **Types**

Palliative care may include medications for pain management, emotional support through counseling, and assistance with end-of-life decisions.

- **Possible Limitations**

Not Curative: Palliative care focuses on symptom management and improving the quality of life but is not intended to cure the underlying cancer.

Resource Availability: Access to comprehensive palliative care services may be limited, depending on the healthcare system and location(Teoli et al., 2023).

7. Clinical Trials

- **How they work**

Clinical trials are research studies that test new treatments or treatment combinations. They offer patients access to potentially groundbreaking therapies that are not yet available to all patients.

- **Types**

There are various phases of clinical trials, and participants are closely monitored for safety and effectiveness.

- **Possible Limitations**

Eligibility Criteria: Clinical trials have specific eligibility criteria, which may limit access for certain patients.

Experimental Nature: The experimental nature of clinical trials means that the effectiveness of the treatment is still being evaluated. There is no guarantee, so the potential risks must be carefully considered.

****

Nothing seemed to work for me. Not to the level I wanted things to work, at least!

They say a phoenix is a mythical creature born from its ashes.

It was about time a phoenix arose from the ashes of all the treatment options I had explored.

Turn over the page; we will now discuss the birth of a protocol!

Chapter 4 - Conventional Oncology - a Success or a Failure?

Overview

Cancer stands as the second major cause of death in the United States, falling only behind heart disease. Despite advancements and a decline in mortality rates since the early 90s', largely attributed to reduced cigarette smoking, the overall progress against cancer seems questionable. Dr. Ian Hains, for example, has challenged the prevailing notion of a victorious "war" against cancer, courtesy of the limitations of the conventional treatment(Haines et al., 2011).

Challenges with Chemotherapy

Take, for example, the aggressive nature of chemotherapy that not only affects cancer cells but also harms rapidly dividing normal cells. This leads to side effects such as nausea, vomiting, and bone marrow suppression(Gyanani et al., 2021).

Chemotherapy can eradicate the bulk of a tumor, but it often falls short due to the presence of cancer stem cells (CSCs). These are dormant cells that are resistant to chemotherapy and are hidden until they activate later and cause relapse.

Dr. Fang-Yu Du and colleagues found in 2019 that conventional chemotherapy can inhibit tumor growth, but fails to achieve the same effect against CSCs.

Here, testicular cancer serves as an exception; it is one of the few cancers that can be *"cured"* by chemotherapy. In this case, the cancer has cancer stem cells that are more sensitive to chemotherapy than the tumor bulk cells.

Chemotherapy-Induced Aggressivity and Immune Impairment

A major concern with chemotherapy is its potential to make cancer more aggressive. For example, studies from Nature 2019 have indicated that chemotherapy-induced inflammation encourages rapid cancer growth, increased resistance to cell death, enhanced invasiveness, metastatic behavior, and angiogenesis. In short, it is the precursor to creating a chemo-resistant cancer cell type. In addition, this approach can impair the host's anti-cancer immune response. As a result, tumor cells can escape immune detection and eradication.

How We Need to View Cancer

1. Cancer as a Metabolic Disease

The conventional approach towards cancer mostly revolves around genetic mutations and uncontrolled cell growth. However, recent years have seen researchers emphasize the role of altered metabolism in the initiation and progression of cancer. Cancer as a metabolic disease is a concept that challenges traditional views. As a result, innovative avenues for therapeutic interventions are now opening up(Seyfried et al., 2014).

The central idea of the theory is that the malignant transformation is closely linked to dysregulation in cellular energy metabolism. Normal cells generate energy through oxidative phosphorylation; this is a process that takes place within the mitochondria. But as compared to that, the cancerous cells are tilted toward glycolysis. This is a less efficient but faster method of energy production, this happens even in the presence of energy, and the effect itself is known as the Warburg effect(Liberti & Locasale, 2016).

2. Cancer as a Clever & Adaptable Enemy - Warburg Effect

Proposed by Otto Warburg in the 1920s, the Warburg effect proposes that cancer cells favor glycolysis over oxidative phosphorylation. This leads to an increased glucose uptake and lactate production. Today, there exists enough evidence that

42

this metabolic switch is a hallmark of many cancer types. The Warburg effect promotes rapid growth and proliferation.

Warburg effect is not just a consequence of genetic mutations. Instead, it is an adaptation of cancer cells to their microenvironment - read that again!

Thus in my experience and belief, limiting sugar would reverse or prevent this undesirable adaptation. This adaptive process enables cancer cells to meet the high-energy demands that are associated with uncontrolled proliferation. Moreover, metabolic reprogramming brings about additional benefits to cancer cells, which include increased resistance to apoptosis and enhanced ability to invade surrounding tissues.

So what are the key players? Oncogenes and tumor suppressor genes can influence cellular signaling pathways that regulate metabolism. The PI3K/AKT/mTOR pathway is of prime importance and plays a crucial role in coordinating cell growth and metabolism. Dysregulation of this pathway is commonly observed in cancer and brings about glycolysis(Y. Peng et al., 2022).

There is an important point here regarding the Warburg effect. It encompasses a broader understanding of cellular energetics. Here, mitochondria's role in the discussion is important. Dysfunction in mitochondrial metabolism has been implicated in cancer progression(Spinelli & Haigis, 2018).

The implications of the metabolic theory of cancer are profound, especially in the context of therapeutic strategies. This approach provides a unique opportunity for intervention. Because of this discussion, the drugs that inhibit glycolysis or modulate mitochondrial function can be explored as anticancer agents. Then, further interventions such as caloric restriction and ketogenic diets that limit the availability of glucose to cancer cells are becoming more popular as well.

There do exist the distinct metabolic vulnerabilities of cancer cells upon which the success of these treatments exists. It is the nature of cancer cells to become heavily reliant on specific metabolic pathways that serve as a potential target for therapeutic intervention. Precision medicine approaches hold promise for tailoring treatments to exploit these vulnerabilities effectively.

3. **Cancer as a Parasite**

   Cancer's exploration as a parasitic disease unveils an exciting intersection between oncology and infectious diseases. Recent research has delved into the possibility of cancer being influenced or even triggered by parasitic infections. Sounds interesting, right? The modern approaches have challenged cancer etiology and treatment of conventional nature, thereby presenting a unique opportunity for novel therapeutic strategies.

   The idea first emerged at the top when Scottish pathologist William Russell reported the presence of a "cancer microbe" within cancer cells. This was the first early glance at the potential link between microscopic organisms and cancer. This idea, however, was met with skepticism, and subsequent researchers championing this idea were often labeled as medical heretics(Faden, 2016).

   But fast forward to the 21st century, and the notion of cancer as a parasitic disease is experiencing a resurgence. At the 14th Annual International Integrative Oncology Conference in 2016, Dr. Nooshin Darvish

   https://drdarvish.com/glioblastoma-linked-to-lyme-disease/

   presented case reports that added a contemporary dimension to this age-old hypothesis. This case described glioblastoma multiforme patients whose tumors regressed upon treatment for parasitic diseases, specifically targeting the spirochete parasite Borrelia, known for causing Lyme disease. The fact that all tumor samples stained positive for Borrelia further added credence to the fact that parasitic infections might play a role in cancer development.

Further investigation into Borrelia's association with cancer revealed intriguing connections. In 2008, Dr. Claudia Schhopt's research found that patients testing positive for Borrelia antibodies had a significantly higher risk of developing mantle cell lymphoma. This again added more credence to the argument that Borrelia might be a little more intricately linked to cancer than previously thought(Schöllkopf et al., 2008).

Animal models have also contributed to our understanding of the potential parasitic influence on cancer. The Cryptosporidium-induced colon cancer model, studied by Dr. Sadia Benamrou and colleagues in 2014, showed that mice inoculated with the Cryptosporidium parasite unexpectedly developed colon cancer. As a result, researchers decided to focus more on the link between parasitic infections and cancer development(Sawant et al., 2020).

The treatment of cancer patients with antiparasitic drugs by oncologists adds a new twist to the story. Cancer patients, who are often immunosuppressed, are routinely given antiparasitic chemoprophylaxis. This practice can affect a patient's immune response and may affect cancer progression. The delicate balance between eradicating parasitic infections and potentially affecting cancer outcomes raises intriguing questions that the medical world needs to find answers to, very soon. Moreover, of course, the story extends beyond Borrelia and Cryptosporidium to other parasitic infections. Q fever, caused by Coxiella burnetii, has been associated with non-Hodgkin's lymphoma (NHL)(Sawant et al., 2020).

So, what has been done at the molecular level to investigate this? The activation of specific pathways within host cells by parasites has been identified as a potential mechanism driving cancer-like behavior. Take the example of the Theileria annulata study in 2014 that revealed that host cell motility and

45

invasiveness were driven by the activation of the MAPK pathway by the inflammatory cytokine TNF Alpha(Ma & Baumgartner, 2014). Now that opened up a pathway for potential treatments!

In 2019, Dr. Cléa Melenotte's study of acute Q fever caused by Coxiella Burnetii identified changes in gene transcription in peripheral blood monocytes. The inference drawn here was that the infection triggered the expression of genes involved in both apoptotic and proliferative mechanisms, explaining that the process was much more complex than what appears at the surface(Melenotte et al., 2019).

Antiparasitic drugs are quite promising in this context. Nitazoxanide was originally developed as an antiprotozoal drug and emerged as a potent Wnt pathway and IL-6 cytokine inhibitor. The Wnt pathway is crucial in cancer stem cell regulation, and inhibiting it could have profound implications for cancer treatment. Nitazoxanide's suppression of protein disulfide isomerase (PDI), overexpressed in ovarian tumors and other cancers further positions it as a therapeutic agent(Li et al., 2021).

Mebendazole, an anthelmintic, has been repurposed as a potent anticancer agent as well. Its mechanism of action is that it disrupts microtubules, impairs mitotic spindle formation, and prevents cell division. The downregulation of anti-apoptotic proteins like BCL-2 further adds more to its anticancer effects. Researchers are thinking that it can replace the standard chemotherapy drugs, such as vincristine, with Mebendazole. The stories of individuals like Joe Tippens, who reported significant improvements using fenbendazole, a veterinary antiparasitic drug, underscore the potential impact of this paradigm shift(Song et al., 2022).

So, what have we learned so far? The intricate connections between parasitic infections and cancer, observed at clinical, molecular, and therapeutic levels, challenge the conventional wisdom surrounding cancer. In addition, as we unravel the complexities of this relationship, we are one step closer to finding innovative solutions that could revolutionize cancer treatment and improve patient outcomes.

Inching Toward an Alternative Solution – Repurposed Drugs

As the researchers are acknowledging the limitations of conventional chemotherapy, there is a growing call for a massive paradigm shift in oncology.

Drs. Daphne Day and Lillian Siu have argued for a more systematic, high-throughput approach to drug screening. They say that this approach must focus on understanding tumor biology and recognizing novel drug combinations that have a powerful effect.

This is where repurposed drugs have gained attention. These are existing drugs, initially approved for specific purposes, and now used "off-label" for cancer treatment. Some of these drugs include statins, anti-inflammatory medications, and antifungals, repurposed for their anti-cancer potential.

But What are Repurposed Drugs? Never Heard of Them! Oh Wait... We Have!

The following lines explore the potential of repurposed drugs in targeting cancer stem cells (CSCs); the focus is more on mechanisms and effectiveness. Several repurposed drugs are currently in clinical trials for various cancers. The Care Oncology METRICS Study, as of May 2023, involves 207 cancer patients receiving drugs like atorvastatin, metformin, doxycycline, and mebendazole. The METRICS study, specifically focusing on glioblastoma patients, has shown promising preliminary data, nearly doubling survival times(Agrawal et al., 2019).

1. Sulfasalazine

Sulfasalazine, originally designed for inflammatory bowel diseases, demonstrates promise in inhibiting CSCs. Targeting the cysteine/glutamate antiporter system (xCT) hinders cysteine uptake crucial for cancer cell survival(Thanee et al., 2021).

2. Pyrvinium Pamoate

Inhibiting Wnt and Hedgehog Pathways Pyrvinium pamoate, an FDA-approved antiparasitic drug, is a potent anti-CSC agent. It inhibits the Wnt and Hedgehog pathways, displaying efficacy against various cancer types, including breast cancer, glioblastoma, and leukemia. Pyrvinium's unique role extends to the tumor microenvironment. It disrupts NADH fumarate reductase activity, affecting mitochondrial energy production within the tumor microenvironment and presenting a novel therapeutic target(Ahmed et al., 2016).

3. Mefloquine

Potential Stem Cell Agent *Mefloquine*, commonly used for malaria prevention, exhibits potential as a stem cell agent. Its impact on mitochondrial function and accumulation in tumor cells makes it a quite promising candidate(Lundström-Stadelmann et al., 2020).

4. Chloroquine and Megas

Autophagy Inhibitors Chloroquine and Mefloquine are autophagy inhibitors and can be explored for their potential to target cancer stem cells. They can disrupt lysosomal function, and contribute to the overall anti-CSC properties(Goel & Gerriets, 2023).

5. Artemisinin

Synergy with Ferroptosis Inducers Artemisinin, coupled with ferroptosis-inducing agents, shows a potential to target cancer stem cells. The synergy with compounds like artesunate and sorafenib can further promote ROS accumulation and iron-dependent cell death.

The selective action of these drugs on key pathways and interactions with the tumor microenvironment highlights the potential for repurposed drugs in advancing cancer therapies(Chen et al., 2020).

6. **Aspirin**

Aspirin, also known as acetylsalicylic acid (ASA), has a history that dates back to ancient civilizations like the Sumerians and Egyptians. More popularly used for various ailments, it has gained attention as a potential anti-cancer stem cell (CSC) agent. It can act as an anti-cancer stem cell agent by suppressing glycolysis.

- Dr. Yin Cao in 2017 associated long-term aspirin use with reduced cancer mortality. The mechanism involves a decrease in overall mortality, primarily from cancer, emphasizing its potential preventive role. It controls nuclear factor kappa B (NF-KB) and downstream inflammatory factors, such as cyclooxygenase-1 and -2 (COX-1 and COX-2)(Cao et al., 2016).

    https://www.ncbi.nlm.nih.gov/pmc/articles/PMC4900902/

- Research by Dr. Weiguang Feng suggests that aspirin inhibits glycolysis in breast cancer stem cells, specifically targeting pyruvate dehydrogenase kinase (PDK). This disruption leads to a shift from glycolysis to oxidative phosphorylation (OXPHOS), suppressing CSC maintenance(F. Peng et al., 2018).

    https://www.ncbi.nlm.nih.gov/pmc/articles/PMC5851116/

- Aspirin's impact on Voltage-Dependent Anion Channel (VDAC) is explored in a 2017 study. By affecting VDAC, aspirin can disrupt the cancer cell metabolism

49

and induce cell death, providing insights into its potential as an anti-cancer agent(Tewari et al., 2017).

https://pubmed.ncbi.nlm.nih.gov/28327594/

- Similarly, Rajendra Langley's 2015 summary explains Aspirin's role in preventing and treating cancer. Inhibition of CSC dissemination and maintenance, as demonstrated in randomized trials, highlights its effectiveness against malignancy development.

- Dr. Kelvin Tso's study in 2019 explained a significant reduction in various cancers among long-term aspirin users. While breast cancer incidence remains unaffected, other cancers, including liver, stomach, colorectal, and lung, show notable decreases.

https://www.researchgate.net/scientific-contributions/Kelvin-KF-Tsoi-217 4135732

- Research by Dr. Joseph Sung in 2019 indicates that aspirin use post-colorectal surgery is associated with a 31% reduction in colon cancer mortality and a decrease in all-cause mortality(J. J. Y. Sung et al., 2019).

https://pubmed.ncbi.nlm.nih.gov/30515899/

As we have just seen, Aspirin can disrupt cancer cell communication, inhibit inflammation, and modulate the tumor microenvironment, contributing to its anti-cancer properties. Aspirin's multifaceted actions, from glycolysis inhibition to modulation of key pathways make it a promising agent in cancer treatment.

7. Metformin

Metformin is widely known as an effective anti-diabetic drug. It is used for controlling blood sugar levels in type-2 diabetes. Recently, it has gained attention as a potential anti-cancer agent as well(Suissa & Azoulay, 2012). Metformin use is associated with a 23% reduction in cancer incidence; no wonder researchers are trying their best to understand how it works!

The first thing here to understand is how it works. Metformin accumulates inside cancer cells' mitochondria, the microscopic energy-producing organelles. Once inside the mitochondria, Metformin interferes with the electron transport chain, specifically inhibiting complex I. This inhibition leads to a shift in cancer cell metabolism, resulting in increased glucose consumption and lactate production. Here, let us talk about a key player called Hexokinase 2 (HK2), an enzyme that is crucial for the rapid proliferation of cancer cells. Metformin disrupts the interaction between HK2 and the voltage-dependent anion channel (VDAC) on the outer mitochondrial membrane. As a result, mitochondrial apoptosis is triggered, and cells can die, as they should normally(Kasznicki et al., 2014).

- Metformin impairs glucose consumption in cancer cells, reducing FDG (fluorodeoxyglucose) uptake in PET scans. The drug hampers HK2 function, which results in decreased cancer cell growth rates and impaired glucose consumption.
- It induces protective autophagy by inhibiting the mTOR pathway. Metformin-induced autophagy can be a double-edged sword, promoting cell survival or contributing to cell death; it varies from situation to situation.
- Metformin can also target cancer stem cells (CSCs). Since the drug can inhibit oxidative phosphorylation, it becomes important in this context since cancer stem cells rely on OXPHOS for functionality.
- Combining Metformin with autophagy inhibitors, such as chloroquine, can enhance its anticancer effects. The balance between protective and harmful autophagy can be upset a little because of this as well.

- The combined use of Metformin and glucose inhibitors or other metabolic inhibitors can lead to the creation of a lethal environment for cancer cells.
- Metformin has also been linked to epigenetic effects in cancer cells, influencing gene expression patterns. Its role in targeting specific signaling pathways and transcriptional regulators in cancer cells then becomes quite apparent(Kasznicki et al., 2014).

8. Vitamin C

Let us start with Susan's story, a patient who sought hormone replacement for relief from menopausal symptoms. However, a routine sonogram revealed a pelvic mass, prompting further investigation. Subsequent tests confirmed ovarian cancer, which had already spread. Susan underwent laparoscopic surgery, a hysterectomy, and removal of metastatic deposits. Following a swift recovery, she was slated for chemotherapy. Susan's sister recommended Intravenous Vitamin C (ascorbate) as a complementary therapy. However, Susan's oncologist opposed it, fearing a reduction in chemotherapy effectiveness. Contrary to this belief, research over the past two decades demonstrates that high-dose IV vitamin C synergizes with conventional chemotherapy, making it more effective.

So, what does science say?
- Studies, including one by De Chestian Kubacher in 1996, reveal that IV vitamin C can further enhance the antineoplastic activity of chemotherapy drugs like doxorubicin and cisplatin in breast cancer cells(Kurbacher et al., 1996).

https://pubmed.ncbi.nlm.nih.gov/8635156/

- Dr. Jeanne Disko and Dr. Yan Ma have also supported the idea that high-dose ascorbate improves chemotherapy sensitivity while reducing toxicity.

52

- <u>Drs. Michel Gonzalez</u> and <u>Hugh D. Riordan,</u> emphasize that high-dose IV vitamin C is one of the safest and most valuable substances for treating cancer(González et al., 2005).

  <u>https://pubmed.ncbi.nlm.nih.gov/8635156/</u>
  https://pubmed.ncbi.nlm.nih.gov/16570523/

- Certain cancers, such as lymphomas and iron-containing multiple myeloma, show sensitivity to IV vitamin C. Studies highlight its efficacy in inducing reactive oxygen species (ROS) and selectively targeting cancer cells. As a result, the antioxidant system is inhibited and the glycolysis process is inhibited, this makes cancer cells vulnerable to oxidative stress.
- Unlike conventional chemotherapy, IV vitamin C targets cancer stem cells. The mechanism of action includes apoptosis and autophagy.
- Combining IV vitamin C with agents like alpha-lipoic acid (ALA) and quinones further enhances its anticancer effects. Here, we are talking about the electron flux through the mitochondria, which can trigger apoptosis in cancer cells.

One has to consider potential drug interactions, such as with vitamin K and warfarin. These drug interactions can be managed with caution of course

9. Cannabis and CBD

In recent times, the use of cannabinoids from cannabis, particularly Cannabidiol (CBD) and Cannabis Oil has also become quite popular. Today, there exist countless accounts of a personal nature, which suggest its effectiveness in alleviating symptoms. In some cases, it can even affect the aggressive nature of the cancer.

- A 14-year-old diagnosed with Acute Basophilic Leukemia in 2006, reveals instances where families, dissatisfied with conventional treatments, explored the use of cannabis oil. The reported rapid reduction in leukemia progression sparked further interest in the potential of cannabinoids.

- Individuals like <u>Rick Simpson</u> have become advocates for cannabis oil, sharing stories of remission and reduction of leukemia symptoms. The "Phoenix Tears" extract, administered orally, has demonstrated dose-dependent effects in some cases.

  <u>https://karger.com/cro/article/6/3/585/89505/Cannabis-Extract-Treatment-for-Terminal-Acute</u>

- Studies point to CBD oil's role in inducing apoptosis (cell death) and inhibiting cancer cell proliferation, offering promise in leukemia treatment(Seltzer et al., 2020).
- Research by M. Riera in 2015 highlights CBD's ability to induce apoptosis by targeting the voltage-dependent anion channel (VDAC) on the mitochondrial membrane.
- Cannabis's potential across various cancers, including gastric, prostate, breast, lung, and melanoma has been well documented as well.

As attitudes towards cannabis shift, and anecdotal evidence accumulates, the integration of cannabinoids into cancer care prompts a reconsideration of treatment approaches.

10. Antibiotics and Antifungals

Among the many novel strategies that are being currently explored, the use of antibiotics and antifungals in cancer treatment has attracted attention for its potential to address infections, manage treatment-related complications, and even influence the tumor microenvironment. Let us have a look at what has been done in this regard in the following lines. Cancer patients, especially those undergoing chemotherapy, radiation, or other immunosuppressive treatments, are at an increased risk of infections. Infections can interrupt and complicate cancer treatment regimens. Antibiotics and antifungals now have a niche in the oncology setting for their role in managing and preventing these infections.

Antibiotics in the Oncology Setting

Because cancer treatments often weaken the immune system, patients become quite susceptible to infections of various sorts. Antibiotics play a crucial role in preventing and managing bacterial infections, which can range from mild to severe.

However, beyond their role in infection prevention, antibiotics can have a direct and indirect effect on cancer cells. Some antibiotics exhibit anti-cancer properties, they can alter the pathways that are involved in cell proliferation and survival. Take the example of tetracycline and macrolides that have been explored for their ability to inhibit certain signaling pathways that are associated with cancer growth.

Antifungals in the Oncology Setting

Fungal infections can also prove to be particularly problematic for immunocompromised cancer patients. There are antifungal agents, such as azoles and echinocandins that can treat and prevent these infections. There does exist a need for aggressive antifungal therapy with the potential side effects and drug interactions, which often arise in the landscape of cancer treatment.

Antibiotics, Antifungals, and the Tumor Microenvironment

Researchers have tried their best to study this relationship between the microbiome, antibiotics, and cancer. The human microbiome consists of trillions of microorganisms residing in and on the human body. This microbiome often regulates the immune system and influences cancer treatment responses. Antibiotics, by altering the microbiome, may inadvertently affect the tumor microenvironment and treatment outcomes.

However, one has to remember that the use of antibiotics and antifungals in cancer treatment is not without challenges. Antibiotic resistance can limit treatment options and pose a serious threat to public health. The balance that exists between eradicating infections and avoiding unnecessary exposure to antimicrobial agents must be carefully thought about as well.

Conclusion

We have reached the conclusion of this section. In this landscape of cancer treatment, the drugs that we have discussed serve as indispensable tools for managing and treating this disease. Their roles extend beyond their usual roles, with emerging evidence suggesting potential direct and indirect effects on cancer cells and the tumor microenvironment. However, there are challenges, for example, antibiotic resistance and microbiome alterations that can underscore the importance of careful consideration in their use. As research continues to unravel the intricacies of cancer treatment, the integration of these drugs into personalized cancer care holds promise for optimizing treatment outcomes while minimizing complications.

Chapter 5: Birth of a Protocol

The first time I learned about my stage IV cancer, it appeared as if I was descending into uncertainty. Months later, the uncertainty bloomed into an outright nightmare.

The conventional medical treatments had reached their limits to this point. The road ahead looked full of darkness. It is said that often, during these times, we make decisions that can change not just our lives but the lives of others. For me, I was at a point where I had to make a pivotal choice.

Either I could accept my fate as predicted by traditional medicine or explore unchartered territories in search of a remedy that spoke to my body's intrinsic capacity to heal itself.

As you can guess, I took the second option, I knew that I ought to go into the realm of self-devised treatment protocols. It was a journey that reflected not only my desire to survive but also my determination to defy the odds.

****

Quest to Beat Cancer Naturally & Holistically

As you will find later, at the crux of this narrative is the profound transformation that the journey underwent. I placed my faith in conventional medical treatments at first. After all, these protocols were widely accepted due to the promises of modern medicine. But, as time passed, the harsh reality of my situation unfolded. With every passing day, it became apparent that these conventional avenues were failing to produce the results that I desperately sought. It was this need for a fresh approach that became so clear that I started searching for an alternative solution that would complement my body's innate resilience and capacity to heal itself.

My day started with searching for articles in medical literature that might hold an answer to my queries. My evenings were spent studying holistic health books. My nights were dedicated to scientific research that would eventually form the bedrock of my treatment protocol; we will talk about this protocol in detail in the chapters to follow as well.

Where was that remedy? A remedy that would align with my body's natural defenses and help me defeat this deadly disease? The quest drove me to delve into the depths of scientific literature. Academic studies, articles, health publications and books were clustered over my home office. The room resembled a shack of a student trying hard to find answers as fast as he could before the exam because time was running out.

Looking back, I can't help but smile a little. But at the time, it was far from a joyful experience!.

Time was running out and this was no ordinary exam. All would be over soon if I didn't find answers in time!

****

A 360-Degree Shift in Dietary Habits to Starve Cancer

The dietary changes would become an integral part of my self-devised treatment protocol. These changes were nothing short of a culinary and nutritional revolution. To understand the significance of these dietary modifications, I urge you to comprehend the magnitude of transformation they brought into my life. It is at the center of this change to cover the shift from a standard American diet to a keto plant-based regimen. This was a profound change in lifestyle and a strategic approach to shutter cancer's primary fuel source. I was effectively

58

recalibrating my eating habits. I wanted to stay away from the sugar-laden, carbohydrate-enriched foods that were the staples of my diet for years. The dietary shift was not solely about shedding excess weight, rather, it was a deliberate effort to starve the cancer cells of their primary fuel source - glucose!.

Cruciferous vegetables, which comprise staples such as broccoli, cauliflower, kale, and cabbage, emerged as key players in my diary transformation(Ağagündüz et al., 2022).

These cruciferous vegetables are renowned for their remarkable cancer-fighting properties. These foods always presented an opportunity to better equip your body with natural allies that supported innate detoxification mechanisms. This was not just about fighting the cravings, rather, I was making a calculated strategy to enhance my body's defense against cancer.

Vitamin C & Fasting to Weaken Cancer & Fortify Body

Now, couple this with intermittent fasting, which I incorporated into a treatment protocol. This marked another paradigm shift in my diet regimen. Now, this was not sporadic or occasional fasting. Rather, it was a consistent commitment to fasting for at least 16 to 24 hours daily. The significance of extending fasting lies in its capacity to trigger autophagy.

Simply put, autophagy is a natural process through which our body eliminates damaged cells. These modifications were not alone strategies. It was a holistic approach that aimed at strengthening my body and weakening the cancer. The introduction of vitamin C through intravenous administration on fasting days was a testament to the synergy that defined my protocol. This particular facet had dual purposes. Firstly, vitamin C can induce oxidative damage in cancer cells. What it does is that it makes these cells more susceptible to the immune system's assault. Furthermore, it also plays a pivotal role in maintaining my vitality and strength during fasting.

59

The mechanism by which high-dose vitamin C kills cancer cells selectively while leaving normal cells unharmed is a matter of great interest to me. Now, we know that the chemical structure of Vitamin C is similar to glucose. What many people don't know is that in non-primate mammals, glucose is converted to vitamin C by three enzymes in the liver. The final enzyme guano lactone oxidase (GLO) has a mutated gene in primates, explaining why primates (including humans) cannot make their own vitamin C and must acquire it through dietary intake. Vitamin C is avidly taken up into the cancer cell by glucose transporters (GLUT1) and serves as a pro-oxidant, with production of hydrogen peroxide, an oxidant that is toxic to cancer cells since they have reduced levels of the catalase enzyme needed for degradation of hydrogen peroxide. Extracellular spaces and normal cells, however, contain plenty of catalase enzymes, which promptly degrade the hydrogen peroxide, explaining why normal cells are unharmed(Mussa et al., 2022).

****

The bulk of a cancer mass consists of rapidly replicating cancer cells. However, lurking in the mass are a smaller number of CSCS that are dormant, not actively replicating, and are therefore immune to the cell-killing effects of chemotherapy. This explains why chemotherapy treatments may induce a brief remission with a "clean" PET scan. The cancer mass is de-bulked by the cell-killing effects of the chemotherapy, leaving a few CSCS behind to repopulate the cancer mass later on.

*Cancer relapse is usually inevitable after an interval of time, depending on the proliferation rate of the cell type **and in conjunction with dietary and lifestyle causes that remain unchanged**.*

This is why the cancers re-grow and are not cured. Unlike conventional chemotherapy, which is unable to kill CSCs, combination therapy with IV vitamin C attacks the CSCs and may result in complete cure with no further relapse(Ghaffari et al., 2020).

This is just an overview, though. We will talk more about the dietary changes and the protocol in the chapters to come.

****

Well, at this point, I can safely assure you of one thing. The essence of my self-devised treatment protocol is firmly grounded in scientific evidence. It was this scientific evidence that propelled it from a mere experiment into a well-considered strategy that capitalized on the emerging knowledge about cancer's metabolic nature. The dietary choices and lifestyle alterations were not whims. Rather, these alterations were made due to trust in the evolving body of scientific knowledge surrounding cancer metabolism, the role of glucose in uncontrolled cell division, and the potential of supplements in enhancing our body's natural defenses.

Cancer as a Metabolic Disease - A Paradigm Shift

At the center of my protocol was the view that cancer is a metabolic disease. Rather than perceiving cancer as an indomitable adversary, I started recognizing cancer as a condition that was intrinsically linked to my body's metabolic processes. Simply said, it was a seismic shift in the approach to combating cancer. This approach opened up new possibilities and injected optimism in my veins that I desperately needed in the face of this daunting disease(Seyfried & Shelton, 2010).

From the metabolic viewpoint, it became apparent to me that cancer was a disease of modern times, one that primarily results from our food consumption patterns and sedentary lifestyle. The overabundance of food, particularly refined carbohydrates and sugars, and continuous eating, are the principal culprits. This perspective offered me a glimmer of hope and potential in the battle against

61

cancer, giving support to me in my quest for alternative treatments rooted in science and reason(Gyamfi et al., 2022).

Unveiling the Dietary Secrets of Human Evolution: A 200,000-Year Time-Travel

In contemplating cancer from an evolutionary perspective, one can't help but reflect on what food was available to early humans and how accessible it was. The answer was unequivocal—our ancestors subsisted on a diet that was as "organic" as possible. It consisted of fruits, berries, nuts, seeds, insects, and small game. There were no supermarkets, no processed foods, and no refined sugars. Basically, a diet that was intrinsically connected to the natural world, devoid of any artificial additives and excessive sugar which are symbolic of the modern diet.

From this vantage point, the human body was designed to withstand prolonged periods without food. This is a remarkable testament to our body's adaptability and resilience. Our forefathers extended periods of fasting that were driven by the necessity of the hunt or the unpredictability of food sources. For me, this point of view was enlightening and personally transformative, this line of thinking helped me make informed the dietary choices that would shape my treatment protocol.

I translated this evolutionary perspective into actionable strategies for combating cancer. I started to see cancer in a new light—a reflection of a modern metabolic disease that was fueled by our detrimental eating habits. I now sought to confront cancer's uncontrolled cell division by interrupting the primary source of its energy—glucose.

Cancer cells, with their rampant and uncontrolled cell division, require a substantial amount of energy. To sustain their rapid growth, they need ample amounts of glucose. By pursuing a new dietary strategy, I aimed to starve these cancer cells by reducing sugar and glucose intake to minimal levels. By cutting off their primary source of fuel, glucose, I sought to cripple their capacity to thrive and multiply.

****

However, cancer is a many-headed monster, one that is an adaptable adversary capable of switching to alternative energy sources when faced with a glucose shortage. I recognized this adaptability and addressed it through the strategic inclusion of supplements that would block potential metabolic pathways that cancer cells might exploit to use glutamine also. Researchers like Dr. Thomas Seyfried, argue

(https://www.ncbi.nlm.nih.gov/pmc/articles/PMC3941741/

that disrupting these metabolic pathways could significantly hinder cancer growth, and it was this line of research that interested me a lot.

Supplements played a pivotal role in the comprehensive strategy that was taking shape. Substances like quercetin, berberine, and curcumin have been used for centuries in various traditional healing systems. These supplements had a history of coexistence with humans, and their safety and efficacy were well-documented in scientific literature. Today, they are finding a new place in the battle against cancer.

Vitamin C, which is a seemingly ordinary nutrient found in fruits like oranges and lemons, has emerged as a potent ally in the fight against cancer. Oxidative damage to cancer cells can render them more visible to the immune system, which could then more effectively target and eliminate these rogue cells. Research by Linus Pauling,

https://www.cancer.gov/research/key-initiatives/ras/news-events/dialogue-blog/2020/yun-cantley-vitamin-c a Nobel laureate, demonstrated the significant potential of intravenous high-dose vitamin C in cancer treatment.

****

Feast & Famine: Navigating Intermittent Fasting

Fasting played a pivotal role in my protocol. A proposed mechanism suggests that fasting induces a state of metabolic stress, a transformation that eventually leads to changes in cellular processes. Simply speaking, it is these cellular processes which could selectively make cancer cells more vulnerable to treatment. Researchers also believe that fasting may reduce the levels of certain growth factors and hormones. This reduction eventually leads to creation of an environment that is less conducive to cancer cell proliferation.

If you are someone who is bent on putting their faith in the traditional cancer treatments, fasting can mitigate some of the side effects associated with cancer therapies. A temporary reduction in nutrient availability can potentially protect normal cells from the harmful effects of treatment. It is understood that it is crucial for cancer patients to undertake fasting under the guidance of healthcare professionals.

Beyond the immediate benefits of weight loss, it triggered autophagy, a process by which the body eliminates damaged cells during periods of fasting. In essence, it was a biological mechanism that favored the survival of the fittest, ensuring that only the healthiest cells endured. In the context of cancer, this process was particularly significant. Cancer cells, with their damaged DNA, were particularly susceptible to autophagy, making this innate cellular process an invaluable asset in the battle against this relentless disease.

The individual responses to fasting can vary, and hence, the approach has to be a careful one, especially with reference to the patient's overall health and specific cancer type. While more research is needed to establish the full extent of fasting's benefits for cancer patients, the preliminary findings are suggestive of the fact that it holds promise as a complementary strategy to conventional cancer treatments.

****

Curcumin - Harnessing the Golden Spice's Power Against Inflammation and Oxidative Stress!

And then somewhere in my diet, I had to add curcumin. It was as simple as that.

Curcumin is isolated from turmeric and has a two-thousand year history of medicinal use as an antioxidant, anti-inflammatory, antimicrobial, anti-carcinogenic, thrombus-suppressive, hepatoprotective, cardiovascular-protective, neuroprotective, and anti-arthritic. A massive body of scientific evidence on curcumin shows this natural plant substance kills CSCS while sparing normal cells. The food spice, curcumin (turmeric) is widely available as a nutritional supplement and targets CSCS(Giordano & Tommonaro, 2019).

In 2016, Dr. Y. T. Huang found in his research that curcumin induces apoptosis of colorectal cancer stem cells by coupling withCD44 Marker(Huang et al., 2016). Dr. Huang and colleagues studied colorectal CSCs and found curcumin couples with the CD44 CSC membrane marker and blocks cell uptake of glutamine, inducing apoptosis in the CSC. The researchers proposed that curcumin might have some blocking effect on the transport of glutamine into the cells, thus decreasing the glutamine content in the CD44+ cells and inducing apoptosis.

A combination of curcumin and epigallocatechin gallate from green tea (EGCG) can inhibit CSCS via down regulation of STAT3-NF-kB signaling. The CSC marker CD44+ protein decreased following treatment of the cancer cells with curcumin and EGCG.

65

In 2012, Dr. Zainul Hasanali et al. studied curcumin in a B-cell lymphoma (mantle cell) model, finding that curcumin inhibits nuclear factor kappa B (NF-KB) activation and down regulates cyclin D1, thereby inducing apoptosis. There was synergy with bortezomib, a new protease inhibitor drug used for hematologic malignancies.

Curcumin also inhibits NF-kB activation, induces cell cycle arrest at the G1/S-phase, and induces apoptosis in mantle cell lymphoma(Shishodia et al., 2005). The expression of all NF-kappa-B-regulated gene products are downregulated by curcumin leading to the suppression of proliferation, cell cycle arrest at the G1/S-phase(Huang et al., 2016).

****

As you can see the synergy between scientific understanding and my protocol was profound, it was a blend of rigorous research with a personal journey of transformation and hope. My approach was grounded in the belief that by equipping my body with the right tools, I could start the process of healing. I incorporated these scientifically-backed dietary and lifestyle modifications to exploit the inherent vulnerabilities of cancer. Rather than pitting my body against harsh treatments like traditional chemotherapy and radiation, I aimed to harness its innate healing potential.

****

Chapter 6: The Power of Supplements

My Hopes Start Getting Up

If you have played video games, you will know that even the best warrior characters can only win battles if they fight with the right tools.

In my battle against cancer, it was the same too. I needed the right tools, or in this case, the potions that would heal my battle-fatigued body. That is where the supplements came into play. Such was the power of the supplements and their impact on my battle against cancer that I decided to dedicate an entire chapter to these supplements. Every supplement that I chose was nothing but a beacon of hope in my relentless pursuit of survival.

The supplements I chose were not randomly selected. Instead, they were selected after meticulous research, a deep understanding of their scientific significance, and their potential to offer hope to those battling cancer. The synergy of these supplements worked well in harmony with the pharmaceutical component of my protocol and resulted in significant tumor regression.

As I have been maintaining since the beginning, this is not just a recap of my journey but a journey others can embark on. *I am just a messenger of hope, that is all!*

****

The Six Steps of Success

The idea behind these supplements and food choices had many objectives. Before I discuss all of the supplements and share their brief profile, plus the scientific rationale behind using them, I think I should share the six successful steps over cancer. Here is how I went about this whole affair.

1. The first step was to starve the cancer of glucose: Cancer cells rely heavily on glucose as their primary fuel source. Therefore, if I could succeed in reducing or eliminating sugar and glucose from my diet, I would be able to create an inhospitable environment for cancer cells.

2. My next step is to block the alternate pathways. Since cancer cells are adaptable, they can switch to alternative energy sources. The supplements I selected have the potential to block these metabolic pathways and further starve the cancer. Hence, opting for these supplements was quite an easy choice for me(Keenan & Chi, 2015).

3. Inhibiting angiogenesis is a crucial step when one is battling cancers at such an advanced stage. By obstructing the formation of new blood vessels that were practically feeding the tumors, I could cut off this sort of supply line, leaving the cancer cells in a starved and weakened state. This is where the modern targeted therapy Cabozantinib played a role(Adair & Montani, 2010).

4. Oxygenate and increase hemoglobin would be the following mantra. Oxygen is our body's primary aid in the natural defense processes, and if I could optimize its availability, I could do something great here. The higher the hemoglobin levels were in my body, the higher the oxygen for my cells and the lesser the cancer. If oxygen levels are low in the blood, it causes hypoxia which triggers more blood vessels to grow in the cancer tumors thus feeding them(Pittman, 2011).

5. After researching the immune system's working and function carefully, I decided to strengthen my immune system, something that would not have been possible had I opted for traditional chemotherapy and radiation treatments. Now, looking back, not opting for traditional chemo was the best thing I did!

6. The protocol that I designed for myself leveraged my body's innate ability to heal and protect itself against different kinds of cancer. Autophagy, the process of cells eating damaged cells, became one of my primary tools against cancer, which is triggered during fasting. Specifically prolonged fasting typically more than 16 hrs studies suggest..

68

<u>Vitamin C (Ascorbic Acid), You Are My Best Friend!</u>

A lot of us think that vitamin C is the perfect remedy for the common cold. Yes, that is true. But in my case, it was destined for a far more profound role. I always passed by Vitamin C supplements in the pharmacy and very rarely invested in them. *Now, things were going to change.*

The scientific rationale for including high-dose <u>IV vitamin C</u> in my protocol was well established. The two-time Nobel laureate <u>Linus Pauling</u> has well-established vitamin C's importance in the fight against cancer.

https://www.nobelprize.org/prizes/peace/1962/pauling/facts/

<u>My superhero move was administering IV Vitamin C while on my 48 hr fast as previously discussed.</u>

Pauling's research opened a new avenue of research. It showed us that IV vitamin C can potentially inflict oxidative damage on cancer cells. Once these cancer cells are damaged, they become super vulnerable to our body's immune system. Think of it this way: our body can identify and eliminate these rogue cells. This research elevated vitamin C from a simple nutrient to a critical weapon in the battle against cancer. From my research, vitamin C has to be administered via IV in order to reach therapeutic levels in the bloodstream.

My super hero move is to administer IV Vitamin C while fasting at least 16hs and remain on the fast for 48 hrs. Of course, one has to build up to this length of time and with the guidance of your doctor.

Quercetin: My Shield against Angiogenesis

To some, quercetin is a unique compound, a flavonoid that is unheard of. However, in reality, it is found in everyday foods like onions, apples, and berries. Quercetin also became a formidable asset in my battle against cancer. Research studies have already established that quercetin is a powerful antioxidant, and it can potentially hinder angiogenesis. Angiogenesis refers to the formation of new blood vessels, vessels that feed our tumors(Xu et al., 2019).

One of the primary objectives in the fight against cancer is to cut off the supply lines. One has to restrict the tumors from accessing the nutrients they desperately require, and this is something quercetin does quite efficiently. You can understand precisely why quercetin became a sentinel in my regimen. It was my guardian angel against the sinister growth of blood vessels that fueled the raging adversary within my body.

****

Berberine: My Lieutenant in Command

Berberine is an alkaloid found in plants such as goldenseal. This compound was initially rooted in traditional medicine, but it has emerged as an effective aid in the modern-day battle against cancer. The science behind Berberine's potential is as compelling as it is cutting-edge. Berberine can interfere with the signaling pathways that perpetuate the survival of cancer cells. You can think as if this compound is a spy with the blueprints to infiltrate the inner workings of the enemy; it similarly dismantles the cancer(Singh et al., 2019).

****

Turmeric with Bioperine: My Golden Guardians!

If we go deep down into history and read in-depth about the evolution of cancer treatment, turmeric, with its active component curcumin, will always find a hallowed place in the annals of history. After I learned all that I needed to learn about turmeric, it was no longer just another spice in the kitchen for me. Instead, it became my guardian against inflammation and a potent antioxidant in my protocol. For curcumin, the scientific understanding went beyond general health benefits. I learned how curcumin could impede the growth of cancer cells, thwart the progression of tumors, and, in some instances, bring about the death of these aberrant cells(Fernández-Lázaro et al., 2020).

Why Bioperine, you may ask. Well, curcumin's potency is often limited by its poor bioavailability, and that is where Bioperine, derived from black pepper, can help massively in the curcumin's strength.

****

AHCC - an Ally of Immunity

Active Hexose Correlated Compound (AHCC) is derived from shiitake mushrooms. In recent times, it has emerged as a crucial ally in the battle against cancer. It provides massive support to the immune system; not only does it bolster the human body's natural defense mechanisms, but it also keeps one in good spirits, courtesy of its overall nutrient profile. Stuff that was vital for me in my quest to conquer cancer.

Scientific evidence supports AHCC's role in stimulating natural killer (NK) cell activity as well. For the sake of simplicity, you can think of the NK cells as the body's specialized assassins trained to identify and eliminate cancer cells. As I added AHCC, my immune army was bolstered, and I felt in a much better position to take on the cancer(Shin et al., 2019).

****

An Ode to Omega-3 Fish Oil

When we think of omega-3 fatty acids, we often picture them as the perfect remedy for inflammation in our body. However, omega-3 fish oil in my protocol had much more importance than serving as a nod to the general well-being.

The scientific rationale for including omega-3 fish oil is, of course, the fact that it can reduce inflammation. However, inflammation also happens to be a process that is closely entwined with the growth and progression of cancer. And in the complex fabric of cancer's survival, omega-3 fish oil was the calming balm I needed to tame this raging storm of inflammation that was raging inside my body(D'Eliseo & Velotti, 2016).

****

Coenzyme Q10 (CoQ10): The Revitalising Force I Needed!

CoQ10 was not just another antioxidant; it was an energetic ally in my battle against cancer. This naturally occurring antioxidant played a central role in the production of cellular energy, a function that made it indispensable in the face of a formidable adversary.

Scientific understanding underscored CoQ10's role in enhancing the body's energy production. This, in turn, bolstered my overall vitality, ensuring I had the resources to endure the trials of the journey ahead(Saini, 2011).

****

Alpha Lipoic Acid: The Armor against Oxidative Stress

Oxidative stress is a potent weapon wielded by cancer. However, Alpha lipoic acid, renowned for its antioxidant properties, stepped forward in these troubled times for me, waving a shield against this monster. The scientific significance of Alpha Lipoic Acid lies in its potential to mitigate oxidative stress and enhance the body's defense mechanisms against various ways cancer progresses in the human body. It's a handy addition to my protocol(Rezaei Zonooz et al., 2021).

****

The Aromatic Avenger and the Immune Guardian

You have guessed it right already, it is garlic! Garlic is often hailed for its distinctive aroma and flavor in culinary traditions. However, for me, it was not just a flavor enhancer; it was a potent force against cancer. During my research on different cancer theories and treatments, I realized the true potential of garlic, that it could hinder the growth of cancer cells. Garlic has many essential compounds; one such active key compound is allicin, a formidable guardian against the cancer onslaught(Zhou et al., 2022).

Zinc - Immune System Boosting Agent

And there was zinc. Ah, it was no ordinary mineral; it was no ordinary mineral for me. Zinc, as some of you may already know, is essential for the development and functioning of immune cells, and immune cells are essential for fighting cancer. Quick math: zinc worked like a charm for me(Dhawan & Chadha, 2010)!

****

Gather, My Fans of Fenbendazole!

Fenbendazole is a benzimidazole drug used to treat different types of cancers. It may prevent carcinogenesis by reducing the proliferation of normal and cancer cells, decreasing the formation of related cancer oncogenes, and blocking the binding of cancer promoters to DNA(Park et al., 2022).

Since it blocks harmful chemicals that are released by cancer cells, and these chemicals cause damage to healthy cells, it is considered to be a helpful agent in the battle against cancer. Cancer cells also make too many proteins called

73

proteases that destroy DNA. Fenbendazole stops the proteases from doing this damage(Dogra et al., 2018).

****

Golden Milk

How can I forget the aromatic concoction that I whipped up for comfort but was also beneficial for my health? I called it Golden Milk, an elixir made from organic almond milk, turmeric, cinnamon, MCT oil, black pepper, cocoa powder, and ground flaxseed.

https://www.healthline.com/nutrition/golden-milk-turmeric#TOC_TITLE_HDR_3

Turmeric, with its anti-inflammatory properties, was the star, and MCT oil and flaxseed added depth to its potency. Black pepper played a crucial role in enhancing turmeric's bioavailability.

****

So, what are the key takeaways from this chapter? One, use natural supplements and foods as much as possible, for they are enriched with nutrients not readily available in a pill. The supplements I chose featured substances that had been around for thousands of years, and at this point in history, our body has adapted to them well enough. And the best part is that the side effects were minimal because our body has already adapted well enough to them. There are different kinds of supplements available in the market, but the ones you should be investing in are the ones with minimal side effects!

Chapter 7 - Sharing the Protocol

Motivation to Share

It is time for me to spill the beans, but before I spill the beans, let me share why I am spilling the beans.

It is like this – imagine you are stuck in a big, wild forest. Out of sheer luck, you suddenly stumble across a map. A map that will show you the way out of the forest.

That is what this protocol is for me.

Therefore, now that I found my way out, I am telling everyone *"Hey, there's a path here!"*

The Protocol

Dietary Foundation: Organic Keto Plant-Based Cruciferous Diet & Fasting

Cancer cells have a sweet tooth, a statement that sounds funny but isn't really. Cancer cells have fifteen times more glucose receptors than normal cells(Adekola et al., 2012). My objective was to starve the cancer cells of its primary fuel source. The organic keto plant-based cruciferous diet helped me cut off the sugar supply. Cruciferous vegetables, rich in anti-cancer properties, assumed a more important role than ever(Higdon et al., 2007).

In order to get my ample supply of nutrient rich cancer fighting foods I ate large salads daily. My salad base was organic spinach, kale and mixed greens. I added celery, grape or cherry tomatoes, raw broccoli, brussel sprouts, cauliflower, mushrooms, cucumber, raw beets, and other low to no sugar vegetables (see list page 145). Eventually, I added boneless and skinless no hormone and no steroid chicken tenders cooked in a cast iron skillet with a little olive oil.

Couple this with fasting, and it is a beautiful combination! Fasting induces autophagy – we have talked about it at a length!

Anticancer Vitamins in Daily Organic Celery-Based Juice

On a daily basis, I was chugging down forty-eight ounces of organic celery-based juice (SUJA brand Uber greens juice). Why celery, you might ask? The reason is that it is a powerhouse of anticancer vitamins. Additionally, it is low in sugar relative to other juices and has vitamin C and K among others. It also contains compounds like apigenin and luteolin. These compounds are known best for their anti-inflammatory and antioxidant properties(B. Sung et al., 2016).

Natural Foods & Substances: Blocking Glutamine Uptake from Cancer Cells

I was not focusing only on supplements. I also worked on incorporating natural foods and substances which I thought would aid me in the fight. I was not looking to attack only cancer cells, but to protect normal cells. Blocking glutamine uptake from cancer cells proved to be a good move. Glutamine is like fuel for cancer, and as its supply diminished because of my actions, I was able to achieve my objectives(Jiang et al., 2019).

Here is a look at some of the fruits that you can consider adding in your diet!

Fruits	Avocados, Strawberries, Blueberries, Raspberries
Vegetables	Arugula, Asparagus, Bell Peppers, Bok Choy, Broccoli, Brussels Sprouts, Cabbage, Cauliflower, Celery, Cucumbers, Eggplant, Garlic, Green Beans, Kale, Lettuce, Mushrooms, Onions, Spinach, Squash, Tomatoes, Turnips, Zucchini
Protein	Salmon, Tuna, Sardines, Trout, Chicken, Turkey
Oils	Flaxseed Oil, MCT Oil
Others	Guacamole, Salsa, Sauerkraut, Pickles, Almonds, Brazil Nuts, Hazelnuts, Walnuts, Macadamias, Olives, Seaweed

Supplement Arsenal: A Detailed Breakdown

Finally, I would like to give this detailed breakdown by not only mentioning the names and amount, but also the rationale and mission behind the usage.

First, let us have a look at the supplements that formed the basic framework of "The Protocol"..

Vitamin D (5,000 IU 3x a day):

- I took vitamin D (5000 IU) thrice a day.
- *Rationale:* I wanted to boost the immune system.
- *Mission:* Keep my defense system strong against the cancer showdown.

Organic Garlic Capsules - Immune System Booster (1,200mg 2x a day):

- *Rationale:* Again, I wanted to boost the immune system.
- *Mission:* Fortification of body defenses.

Turmeric (Curcumin) with Bioperine (1,300 mg 2x a day):

- I took turmeric with bioperine (1300 mg) twice a day.
- *Rationale:* Glycolysis inhibition, anti-inflammatory, VDAC inhibition, mTOR inhibition – activates autophagy, anti-angiogenesis. That is plenty of motivation right there!
- *Mission:* What does doing all of that achieve? Reduction in inflammation, hinder cancer's energy supply, as well as disrupt the growth and survival strategies.

CoQ10 (100 mg 3x a day):

- I took CoQ10 (100 mg) thrice a day.
- *Rationale:* Cardiac and immune system protection.
- *Mission:* Protecting the heart during challenging treatments as well as enhancing overall immune function.

Garcinia Cambogia (800 mg 3x a day):

- I took garcinia cambogia (800 mg) thrice a day.
- *Rationale:* Reduce blood sugar levels.
- *Mission:* Starve the cancer cells by controlling their primary fuel source – sugar.

Green Tea Extract (500 mg 3x a day):

- I took green tea extract (500 mg) thrice a day.

- *Rationale:* Not only does it take care of inflammation, it also prevents chronic conditions like heart disease, diabetes, and certain other forms of cancer.
- *Mission:* The extract can work against inflammation and battle chronic diseases.

Quercetin (500 mg 2x a day):

- I took quercetin (500 mg) twice a day.
- *Rationale:* Quercetin can lead to glycolysis as well as angiogenesis inhibition.
- *Mission:* It blocks cancer's energy production. It also blocks the formation of new blood vessels that feed the cancer cells.

Berberine + Ceylon Cinnamon (625 mg 2x a day):

- I took ceylon cinnamon and berberine (625 mg) twice a day.
- *Rationale:* Anti-inflammatory, cancer stem cell agent.
- *Mission:* Put out inflammation fires, attack the cancer stem cells.

Zinc (50 mg 1x a day):

- I took zinc (50 mg) once daily.
- *Rationale:* Immune system booster.
- *Mission:* Strengthen the immune system elements.

AHCC (500 mg 2x a day):

- I took AHCC (500 mg) twice a day.
- *Rationale:* Betaglucans, they can enhance the anti-tumor immunity.
- *Mission:* Strengthen the immune system's anti-tumor defenses.

Fenbendazole (250 mg 3x per week - M W F):

- I took fenbendazole 250 mg thrice a week.
- *Rationale:* Inhibits cancer cell growth, disrupts microtubial formation in cancer, inhibits glucose uptake.
- *Mission:* Stop cancer cells from growing as well as interrupt their sugar supply.

Alpha Lipoic Acid (300 mg 3x a day):

- I took alpha lipoic acid (300 mg) thrice a day.
- *Rationale:* Glycolysis inhibition, induces apoptosis.
- *Mission:* Disrupt cancer's energy production and trigger natural cell death.

Vitamin C (Liposomal) Capsule (1,700 mg 5x a day):

- I took vitamin C capsules (1700 mg) five times a day.
- *Rationale:* maintain vitamin C in my system in between IV administration.
- *Mission:* Apply stress on cancer cells to weaken them.

Vitamin C IV (25,000 mg 1x per week):

- I took vitamin C IV (25,000 mg) once a week while on min 16 hr fast (48 hr fast if possible).
- *Rationale:* Induces oxidative stress.
- *Mission:* Administer a massive dose of Vitamin C to hit cancer hard.

K2 (100 mg 3x a day with Vit C, also taken on days when administering Vit C IV):

- I took K2 (100 mg) thrice a day with vitamin C therapy.
- *Rationale:* Increases Vitamin C efficacy.

- *Mission:* Team up with Vitamin C to make it extra effective.

Melatonin (30mg/day 10mg am & 20mg pm):

- I took melatonin twice daily.
- *Rationale:* SCOT inhibitor and angiogenesis inhibitor.
- *Mission:* Team up with Cabozantinib and stop cancer growth.

Coley's Toxin (2ul 2 x per week) : (Please note, I obtained Coley's from clinic in Mexico)

- I took Coley's Toxin 2ul two times per week - once while fasting and same day with IV VIt C. Basically, this is a combination of Streptococcus pyogenes and Serratia marcescens.
- *Rationale:* Increases white blood cell activity to help detect and attack cancer cells. The theory here is that bacterial infections can activate the immune system, causing it to produce various immune cells and substances that not only fight the infection but also targetcancer cells.
- *Mission:* Team up with Vit C and hit cancer hard.

Time	8 AM	4 PM – After Meal	10 PM
Vitamin D- 5000 IU	★	★	★
Turmeric With Bioperine- 1300 mg	★		★
CoQ10- 100 mg	★	★	★
Garcinia Cambogia- 800 mg	★	★	★
Green Tea Extract 500 mg (ECGC)	★	★	★
Quercetin- 500 mg	★		★
Berberine + Cylon Cinnamon- 625 mg	★		★
Zinc-50 mg		★	
AHCC-500mg	★		★
Fenbendazole-250mg- 3 X Week- Monday, Wednesday, Friday		★	
Vitamin C Capsule 1700 mg 5 X Day - Vitamin C Total 8500 mg/day	★	★	★
Vitamin C IV- 1 week on a fast			
K2 100 mg- Administer with Vitamin C	★	★	★
Omega 3 Fish Oil 1175 mg	★		★
Melatonin 10mg (30 mg day) Take 20 mg at Bed Time	★		★ ★

Supplement Synergy and Cabozantinib

The main point of this theory lies in the synergy between these supplements and my Cabozantinib pill. Cabozantinib is the leader of the pack. It coordinates and amplifies the effects of each member(Abdelaziz & Vaishampayan, 2017). This combination, along with some very pinpointed lifestyle changes, basically gave me the current results. Results that eventually proved to be a testament to the power of a well-thought-out plan!

Guiding Principles Behind the Actions:

1. **Starve the Cancer of Glucose:**
   - *Rationale:* Cancer cells crave sugar, and by cutting off this supply, we could weaken their growth.

2. **Block Alternate SCOT Enzyme Pathway with Melatonin:**
   - *Rationale:* This was done in order to reduce an alternate energy source for cancer cells(Kassovska-Bratinova et al., 1996).
   - *Mission:* Make sure cancer cells do not have a backup fuel.

3. **Attack and Block Cancer Cells Angiogenesis (Cabozantinib Rx):**
   - *Rationale:* No new vessels that would feed cancer cells!
   - *Mission:* It was just like cutting off the supply lines.

4. **Oxygenate and Increase Hemoglobin in Blood:**
   - *Rationale:* Enhance oxygen supply, a fact that is so crucial for overall health.
   - *Mission:* Create an aerobic environment where cancer cells are not able to survive.

5. **Boost White Cell Activity and Count (AHCC Supplement):**
   - *Rationale:* Fortify the immune system's frontline soldiers.
   - *Mission:* Make sure there is a robust defense in place against cancer.

6. **Strengthen Immune System, Not Weaken It Like Traditional Chemo and Radiation:**
   - *Rationale:* Maintain the human body's natural defense system.
   - *Mission:* Immune system and elements must be in order so that they can fight cancer.

7. **Cause Autophagy (IF and Fasting):**
   - *Rationale:* Turn on the switch for cellular cleanup.
   - *Mission:* Get rid of the damaged cancer cells.

8. **Cause Apoptosis (Natural Cell Death):**
   - *Rationale:* Bring about the natural death of cancer cells.
   - *Mission:* Get rid of the cancer cells naturally.

9. **Use Natural Supplements and Foods as Much as Possible:**
   - *Rationale:* One has to minimize harm to normal cells while at the same time targeting cancer.
   - *Mission:* This would help me maintain a holistic and gentle approach to healing.

10. **Use Targeted Gamma Knife Radiation:**

    - *Rationale:* One has to minimize harm to normal cells while at the same time targeting cancer, especially when it can affect vital organs.
    - *Mission:* Prevent cancer from affecting immediately critical areas.

****

Three Years of Trial and Error

Did I design this protocol in one day? Absolutely not. Rather, it is the result of approximately three years of trial and error, fine-tuning, and observing my body's responses. Tumor regression or elimination in all areas (~12 areas with tumors or enlarged lymph nodes) was the outcome for me, and can be the same for you, diligence and patience is the key! Here are some basic tips in this regard:

- *Make sure you are not munching past 9 PM.*
- *First meal for the next day has to be after 12 noon.*
- *48 oz of green celery-based juice every day- I would say it is a MUST!*
- *1 or 2 meals a day within an 8-hour window*

- *Fill your diet with organic plant-based goodies and a bit of wild-caught fish.*
- *Eventually I added organic chicken*
- *Drink plenty of filtered high pH water*
- *Fast 48 hrs weekly*

There can be slight modifications in this protocol, but essentially, the basic framework will remain the same for you to battle cancer! Remember - NO ADDED SUGAR - Think Keto!

Empathy in Every Step

When someone is fighting cancer, it is not just a physical thing; rather, it is a heart and soul thing too. I have been through enough scary moments, the feeling of lost moments, and the lonely moments. I wandered through this dark tunnel all on my own. Now, sharing it feels like the only right thing to do.

I have been there, and here is a hand to help you out too.

This protocol thing is not just a set of rules. I would like you to think of it as a well-thought, super-smart answer to the struggles I faced. Cancer can make you feel weak as if you have no control. Nevertheless, this protocol is your chance to take some of the lost power back very quickly. So, if my tough times can turn into a way for someone else to find a bit of ease, why keep it to myself?

****

Philosophy behind the Protocol

I am a strong admirer of the human body's innate wisdom. Our body was designed to withstand tough times, and yes, this includes periods when food isn't readily available - FASTING! I wanted to explore that natural resilience and I did that by deploying targeted modern therapies, natural substances, mindful food choices, and strategic fasting.

The idea here? Starve and attack the cancer!

I think that at this point, all of my readers must understand the underlying philosophy steering the course. Nothing too complex, just a thoughtful approach that is rooted in a pragmatic set of principles.

Let's expand a little more on my philosophy

Nature's Wisdom in Healing

At the heart of this philosophy is a deep appreciation for the healing capacity inherent in nature and our own bodies!

It is for the inherent wisdom of nature, the very nature of the human body that is designed in such a manner that promotes healing. Our body possesses a fundamental ability to revitalize and protect itself. This protocol works well with nature's offerings – plants, fish, or ancient remedies – and I have tried to harness the potential of all these offerings. These are the very tools nature has provided us throughout generations for healing; this protocol has employed them in our collective fight against cancer.

Balancing Act: Helping, Not Hurting

When we talk about the cancer treatment landscape, it is often all about aggressive interventions.

However, the philosophy behind this protocol assumes a different stance.

The protocol seeks a delicate equilibrium, a point at which the intervention supports the body's healing mechanisms, while trying to minimze stress and work in conjunction with the body. This mantra is your guide, one that will gently assist your body to combat challenges. It will not overshadow the resilience of the immune system it intends to fortify. The protocol is here to support your body, not to overpower it.

Briefly, the philosophy underpinning this protocol reflects a deep respect for the relationship between nature and the human body. It praises our body's ability to heal when provided with the right resources.

It is time to have a closer look at these resources.

****

Dietary Guidelines: Fueling the Fight

Organic Bounty for the Body

The basis of the dietary approach of our protocol lies in embracing an organic plenteousness for the body. Think of it as if you are stocking your body's defense with very skilled natural defenders. In addition, what defenders they are! Cauliflower, broccoli, kale, and a few other nutrient-packed vegetables (see list in appendix). This incorporation aims at providing the human body with the ammunition it needs to fight cancer. Opting for organic translates into no entry for harmful pesticides and maximizes intake of essential vitamins and antioxidants. As a result, an environment where healthy cells thrive and cancer cells die is established. This is your menu that will bolster the body's natural defenses.

Keto Plant-Based: Cutting the Cancer Feast

Picture rendering your diet somewhat Keto as a move that will disrupt the preferred feast for cancer cells. By reducing sugar and carbohydrates, you can essentially change the locks on the cellular buffet, drastically making it less appealing and exciting for cancer cells to indulge. As opposed to deprivation, this is a strategic selection – one that can starve the cancer cells while nourishing healthy cells. Remember, this is all about creating a diet plan that alters the cellular environment, making it less hospitable to the uninvited guests – cancer cells (Tan-Shalaby, 2017). Remember my daily cruciferous based salads - think organic plant based keto!

Fasting Routine: Giving Cells a Break

Intermittent Fasting: A Cellular Reset

Intermittent fasting (IF) refers to an eating habit or pattern that fluctuates between specified periods of fasting and eating. Intermittent fasting is not a harsh discipline but rather a cellular reset. There are different types of intermittent fasting like the 16/8 method, 5:2 diet, eat-stop-eat method, and many others.

It is a widely accepted fact that a healthy dietary intake that is intended to reduce weight can help with fighting cancer-causing mechanisms in the human body. Obesity is a known risk factor for a variety of cancers like breast, colorectal, hepatobiliary, or pancreatic carcinomas.

But how IF helps the human body in fighting malignancies is still under question. However, some of the evidence that researchers have been able to collect suggests that reduced calorie intake and fasting help make cancer cells more sensitive to various chemotherapeutic regimens, moreover, it also triggers autophagy in the human body.

What is autophagy, you may ask?

It is a combination of two Greek words, *auto* meaning self and *phagy* meaning eating. It is a cellular process triggered by various enzymes leading to the degradation and recycling of various cellular components. During autophagy, the cell forms structures called autophagosomes, which engulf damaged unnecessary cellular components, such as proteins, organelles, and other structures. These autophagosomes then fuse with lysosomes, which are cellular structures containing enzymes that break down and digest the contents of the autophagosomes. This process releases building blocks (amino acids, fatty acids, etc.) that can be reused by the cell for the synthesis of new components. It is a key process in maintaining the body's normal hemostatic environment. Triggering autophagy by intermittent fasting helps fight cancer cells by activating their destruction and degradation thus helping with the normal healing process preventing the accumulation of harmful materials and suppressing tumor formation. It also helps with the clearance of intracellular pathogens, like viruses, bacteria, or other pathogens thus helping with the prevention of superadded infections more prone to develop during malignancies (Bhutia et al., 2013).

So coming back to the benefits of IF, another important aspect is that it reduces blood glucose levels and improves the insulin sensitivity of cells, thus triggering the uptake of glucose by cells making it less available for tumor cells to grow and thus hindering their growth.

So, concluding, the potential benefits of IF include better metabolic health, weight reduction, enhanced insulin sensitivity, and less susceptibility to developing infections, but we are still not sure whether it helps in every cancer patient or not or to which extent it helps in fighting malignancies as individual responses to IF may vary. By incorporating intermittent fasting into the routine, the body gains the opportunity to rejuvenate and optimize its cellular functions.

Vitamin C IV: Oxidizing Cancer Cells

Administering High-Dose Vitamin C: Oxidizing Cancer Cells

We are all set for our superhero move, i.e. administering high-dose Vitamin C IV. What makes this a superhero move in the first place is that it is strategically timed during fasting. A surgical strike against cancer cells, if you will.

Picture an oxidative burst that can create damage specifically within cancer cells. Not only does this burst weaken the cells but it also makes them more visible to the immune system. Thanks to this approach, our body's defense forces can easily identify and eliminate cancer cells quite effectively. There does exist a synergy between high-dose IV Vitamin C and fasting; so the approach is quite similar to a planned assault on cancer cells.

Because of this approach, the human body can leverage the body's innate mechanisms to initiate a much more focused response. This intervention helps to launch a synchronized attack on the cellular level that uses the powerful combination of fasting and Vitamin C to boost the human body's defense mechanisms(Pawlowska et al., 2019).

Lifestyle Practices: Moving and Shaking

Daily Walks and Rebounding: Exercise as Medicine

Exercise is not only a somewhat grueling regimen but also a form of medicine. Daily walks and rebounding exercises are quite effective in keeping the entire body system in motion. Walking daily often proves to be a gentle cardiovascular workout. It promotes blood circulation and enhances oxygen delivery to cells. We have talked about the importance of exercise at length in the previous chapters, so I reckon enough inspiration exists for you to put more faith in the power of exercising daily. Walking is a daly exercise I highly recommend and was a cornerstone of my healing journey, truth be told, a must in my opinion!.

Cold Therapy: Putting Cells on Ice

Cold therapy and cancer, sounds like a tad unconventional combination, right? However, what it does is that it subjects cells to controlled stress. Cold therapy is essentially prompting your body cells to adapt and become more resilient. Once you are exposed to harsh environments, it can stimulate adaptive responses within the body. Mechanisms that can enhance cellular defense are activated.

Technically, you are exposing your body to extreme conditions; but more than that, it is about introducing controlled stressors that trigger beneficial physiological responses. Think of cold therapy as a sort of workout for your cells, one that will make them better equipped to face challenges(Espeland et al., n.d.).

Just as a muscle grows stronger with regular exercise, our cells can become more resilient as well when they are exposed to controlled cold stress. All that you are doing is nudging your body into a state of heightened alertness and adaptability!

Celery Juice: The Everyday Elixir

Now, let us discuss the elixir's role in this protocol.

Celery juice.

It is not the latest trend, at least in this context. Rather, celery juice is a nutrient-packed concoction that has a very specific purpose in this treatment protocol. It is low in sugar and is enriched with enough essential nutrients that can act as a health booster.

I want you to imagine this as a daily ritual, an act of nourishing your body with a concentrated dose of vitamins, minerals, and antioxidants. Introducing a manageable yet impactful addition to your daily regimen such as celery juice can prove to be massively helpful in the future. One can also use a celery based low sugar organic cold pressed juice which is what I do to the tune of approximately

48 oz a day. You can juice it yourself as others have done to help themselves beat this disease or I have found a brand that works for me - it is SUJA Uber Greens.

Battle Allies
Medications, Targeted Therapies & Supplements

Cabozantinib: Blocking Cancer's Supply Lines

Let us talk about Cabozantinib.

If fighting cancer is like a chess game, this pill is your knight. It blocks cancer's supply line and acts as a VEGF inhibitor. The pill has the potential to hinder the growth of blood vessels that tumors rely on for sustenance. The tablet is a targeted intervention that has the potential to starve tumors and impede their ability to thrive. Since Cabozantinib can interfere with angiogenesis, it becomes a key player in the protocol's multi-faceted strategy. A very useful addition, if I may say, in any cancer treatment protocol!

Gamma Knife: Attacking Cancer Tumors Directly

Gamma Knife is a targeted radiation that uses multiple laser beams to focus directly on the tumor that can affect vital areas. In my case - the brain! Basically, Gamma Knife is a form of stereo radiosurgery. The process involves using multiple lasers. Only where the lasers intersect is the radiation strong enough to destroy the cancer cells, leaving the surrounding cells minimally affected. The process is non-invasive, which means that there is no need for surgical incisions. A team of neurosurgeons, radiation oncologists, medical physicists, and radiation therapists conduct this operation.

Vitamin Squad: Strengthening Defenses

What we have at our hands is a team of vitamins and supplements that is working together; each member of this team has a very specific role that is well-defined. Quite pertinent to mention here that this team has been very thoughtfully curated, this lineup can bolster our body's defense mechanism without much trouble. From green tea extract that is rich in polyphenols to vitamin D which is imperative for bone health and proper functioning, each element has its significance in the protocol.

Ancient Wisdom in Modern Pills

Turmeric, quercetin, berberine.

A novice might just think that these are the names of some ancient wise men. Well, they are compounds, but their incorporation to battle cancer is quite a wise move. By doing this, you are just tapping into centuries-old knowledge.

Take Turmeric as an example, with its anti-inflammatory properties, it has assumed the role of a medicinal ally in many diseases. Then there is quercetin, which is present in fruits and vegetables and does wonders with its antioxidant prowess. Lastly, there is Berberine, derived from various plants. It brings its antimicrobial and anti-inflammatory attributes to the party.

I think that at some point, humans will sit down and realize that nature has provided us with solutions that stand the test of time. Sometimes, it is not just about embracing the latest fad; rather one can draw inspiration from the rich tapestry of natural remedies too!

****

Guidance on Implementing the Protocol

Baby Steps to Big Changes

When you have a chance to look back at what I have shared with you so far, you will realize that we have come a long way. It may seem like a lot to do, it might overwhelm you. However, at the same time, if you are thinking about baby steps, you will be able to achieve the bigger milestones quite easily. For example, we have been stressing the importance of sugar intake reduction since the very start of this book. However, if you feel that it is almost impossible for you to give up on the sugar intake completely, then you can start gradually. This also goes for fasting. I hardly expect you to fast for 14-16 hours every day. Start with a number that is realistically possible for you. Eventually, these incremental changes will lead to significant impacts over time, making the transition more manageable.

Consultation with Your Team

The practicality of the protocol is solid, but of course, you must consult with your healthcare team before implementing it. After all, they are the most informed individuals who have your medical history and can give you special personalized advice. So, if you share what I have shared with you, discuss your intentions, and work together to ensure it aligns with your overall health plan, I think you will benefit a lot from it. The protocol, while most of it is well thought, is still subject to some minor alteration. It might be the case that a certain element of the protocol will be eliminated while your healthcare team might suggest a few minor alterations. They say that every patient is unique, and by keeping those standards in mind, we must be careful to approach the protocol. Personalization is key.

In short, it is all about tailoring the dietary guidelines, making fasting routines, and systemically supplementing your dietary intake. Only then can this protocol become a harmonious part of your lifestyle.

Monitoring Progress

Monitor your progress; keep track of dietary changes, fasting periods, and supplements. I suggest a journal or spreadsheet to help with this. This will help you to stay accountable as well as provides valuable insights into what works best for your body. Doing this and monitoring your body can prove to be extremely helpful.

Challenges and Countering Challenges

Navigating Challenges in Implementing the Protocol

If you are to follow this protocol in its very essence, then you must understand that it is undoubtedly a journey that will be filled with hope and potential. However, at some point, you might face some challenges. Understanding the very nature of these obstacles and having proactive solutions in place well in advance can prove to be instrumental in empowering individuals to overcome hurdles on their path to recovery.

Let me share some challenges with their possible fixes.

1. Dietary Adjustments

Challenge: If you are shifting to a Keto plant-based diet for the first time in your life in your bid to make your diet loaded with specific cancer-fighting foods, well it might be challenging, it is not everyone's cup of tea that is for sure!

Solution: The best fix for this problem is to start with gradual changes. Introduce one new food element in your diet at a time, play around with recipes, and reach a balance that suits individual tastes. You can also consult a nutritionist to ensure your nutritional needs are met, it is never a bad idea! The key is to eliminate processed foods, added sugars and switch to a *organic keto cruciferous plant based diet*. Remember - think Keto Plant based!

2. Fasting Routine

Challenge: Intermittent fasting can be a daunting task, especially if you are not used to any kind of fasting, let alone fasting for 16 to 24 hours daily or longer periods. Doing intermittent fasting for two whole days a week can be even more mentally and physically challenging.

Solution: Start with shorter fasting periods and then, if your body is nodding in approval, gradually extend your fasting periods. At the same time, please make sure that you stay hydrated and incorporate nutrient-rich, low-calorie foods in your fasting schedule. Once you can develop a rhythm of some kind, you will feel a lot better.

3. Supplement Adherence

Challenge: Managing a wide-ranging supplement regimen that is loaded with pharmaceuticals like those that Cabozantinib can be a daunting challenge, especially from a logistic point of view.

Solution: What you can do is you can develop a schedule for supplements, one that will ensure consistency. You can use digital calendars and schedule planners. In the meantime, you must regularly check and restock supplements to avoid further interruptions. Also, please make sure that you are in regular communication with healthcare providers. I found that my stomach tolerated the supplements better with food in it and eventually became used to them. As an example, I would have a third of the supplements in the morning while still fasting (water fast) and then after my meal I had my second set of supplements and the third later in the evening while I still had food in my stomach. My times were typically 8am, 3pm and 9pm.

4. Lifestyle Changes

Challenge: Integrating every lifestyle change I mentioned earlier might be overwhelming, especially for cancer patients with physical challenges.

Solution: So here is what you can do. You can personalize these practices based on your capabilities. For instance, low-impact exercises are easily replaced by high-impact rebounding, and cold therapy can be performed at an intensity that is suitable for you.

5. Emotional Resilience

Challenge: Navigating a cancer diagnosis and adhering to a comprehensive protocol can take an emotional toll.

Solution: You have to develop and come up with a support system that consists of your friends, family, or support groups. You should regularly engage in activities that bring joy and relaxation. At the same time, you can perform mindfulness practices, such as meditation or counseling, to bolster emotional well-being.

6. Monitoring Progress

Challenge: Consistently monitoring progress can be tiring without a structured approach.

Solution: Use the formula I shared with you earlier!

Conclusion

As I have just shared the finest details of this protocol with you, I want you to see it as a roadmap forged from my battles and victories. Only then, you will be able to dive into a realm where the resilience of the human spirit meets the precision of scientific strategies. And you will realize that with every challenge, there's a solution waiting to be discovered. The best part for you? *I am*

presenting you with solutions that worked for me!

Chapter 8: Movement & Healing

Can you *out exercise* a bad diet?

In most cases, the answer is no.

However, this hardly undermines the importance of exercise. This is precisely the reason why we are going to explore the healing power of exercise,

In the following lines, we will be taking a closer look at exercise routines that can prove to be beneficial for you, and back what I have to say with science that supports the incredible impact of exercise on the journey of cancer patients.

Unveiling the Healing Power of Movement

When a deadly disease like cancer becomes a part of your life, one can easily feel that their body is no longer something that they control. Treatments and medications are right there at the center stage, but there's one critical aspect of all this story that we mustn't overlook, and that aspect is exercise.

Now, exercise is not not just about staying in shape; rather it's about reclaiming a sense of control and vitality in your life. Better, you can think of exercise as a way of taking back your life from the clutches of cancer.

Physical & Emotional Benefits of Daily Walking

When I look back, I think that life for me in the last few months has been a relentless rollercoaster of emotions and experiences. But even during these tumultuous moments, one thing remained constant, which is my commitment to staying active. Even if I only walked to the corner and back, I had to MOVE!

It was not easy, but I did it anyway!

Daily walks became a ritual that I used to look forward to everyday, but it was not like that initially. Like I mentioned - I HAD TO MOVE! For me, the simple act of moving and breathing in the fresh air became super important. It became a reason for me to connect with nature, and this connection played a crucial role in my healing journey.

Walking, to some, may seem like an ordinary activity. But in my eyes, it became my respite. This was my time to reflect, and rightly said, one of the primary sources of physical and emotional well-being for me. In the following lines, I would like to illuminate the nature of these benefits in detail. Additionally, I knew every step would bring me closer to a healthy body and life.

First, let us talk about the physical benefits that I experienced.

- **It helped me significantly in boosting energy levels, and that is not something that can be done easily.** By this time, I am sure that you can appreciate the manner in which cancer treatments often leave you feeling fatigued and drained. Surprising as it may sound to some, it was these walks, which helped me, counteract this fatiguing effect of cancer. This was my natural boost of energy, which allowed me to face each day with a sense of vitality.
- Muscle wasting is one of the most reported side effects associated with cancer treatments. However, daily walks can help you maintain muscle strength and endurance. I mean, at the very least, you will still be able to go about your daily business in the same manner as before, and for a cancer patient, that is some feat.
- Weight management is a major challenge for many cancer patients. Many cancer patients struggle with changes in body weight, sometimes they are gaining and in other instances, losing. But if you indulge in regular walking, you will be able to manage your weight, something that was crucial for my overall well-being.
- Cancer and cardiovascular disorders often go hand in hand. But by the simple act of walking daily, I was supporting my cardiovascular health, and I was very conscious of this fact. It reduced my risk of heart problems, and put my mind at ease with respect to any cardio problems that may emerge during the cancer treatment.

Now for the section that many of you have been waiting for, folks, exercise does help with emotional disturbances.

- The primary goal on the emotional side of things is to make sure that the patient is not feeling too down. Now, cancer brings with it a massive emotional burden. I found that walking allowed me to let go of stress, and this small walk around a park brought a sense of calm to my life. Walking became my moving meditation, the walk time helped me release worries and find the much-needed peace in my life.

- The act of walking stimulates the release of endorphins. Endorphins are the "feel-good" hormones which can counteract feelings of anxiety and depression. Therefore, when I say that my daily walks practically saved me from falling into the clutches of despair, I am not exaggerating at all.

- Sometimes, you need some *me* time to reflect upon things. Just reflect, nothing more. And I found that out while walking, I was able to contemplate my situation, this walking time helped me seek answers and strategies to cope with my diagnosis and treatment. I also made sure to express gratitude during my walks! *I eventually would do my walks while still fasting which I believed helped in the healing process while being detrimental to the cancer tumors.*

- Among many diseases and disorders out there, cancer is probably one disorder that can make you feel powerless. However, walking and taking some time for myself was an act of taking control. This very basic act served as a reminder that I still had the power to make choices; choices, which could affect my well-being positively.

- It helps with insomnia too, you know. Daily walking improved my sleep quality; this was something that my fatigued body desperately sought. This rest period allowed me to rest more soundly, and helped face each day more refreshed.

- Walking also increased my cardio over time and that is a good thing, especially against cancer cells. Cancer cells use sugar primarily through an anaerobic process which is less effective than the normal aerobic oxygen using process.

Typically cancer does not like oxygen and I believe this was critical to my healing and bringing my body back to a normal state of using oxygen for energy generation instead of the less efficient process of using sugar or glucose.

****

Rebounding: Bouncing Back to Health

Incorporating rebounding i.e. bouncing on a mini-trampoline, in your daily life might seem like an unusual addition for cancer patients, right? And I get your surprise, too. However, like many other things that used to surprise me earlier but do not do so anymore, the benefits of rebounding are quite interesting themselves. Here are some of the reasons as to why you might consider adding rebounding in your daily routine.

- One of the key advantages of rebounding is that this activity can stimulate the lymphatic system. The lymphatic system plays a very vital role in eliminating toxins and waste products from our body, which could prove quite toxic otherwise. Now, as compared to the circulatory system, which relies on the heart's pumping action, our lymphatic system depends on muscle movement for lymph circulation. And that is what rebounding brought to the party too.
- Rebounding engages many of our muscles in a gently efficient manner. The up-and-down motion regulates the flow of lymph, thereby aiding in the removal of toxins, cellular waste, and excess fluids. This is something that is extremely beneficial for cancer patients since it can help reduce the overall swelling and the toxic burden on the human body.
- Furthermore, rebounding also ensures that oxygen and nutrients are delivered adequately to the cells, and at the same time, waste is efficiently removed. Overall well-being, and increased energy levels are the result.

- Some of the traditional exercises can be sometimes hard on the joints. Here I speak especially for individuals battling cancer or those recovering from surgery. As compared to the traditional exercises, rebounding is a low-impact activity. It reduces the risk of joint injury, and provides an excellent way to engage in physical activity without causing too much strain on the human body.
- It is a matter of common observation that cancer and its treatments can affect balance and coordination of the victim. This increases the risk of falls and injuries. But if rebounding is introduced gently, it challenges these faculties, and has the ability to improve the balance and coordination over time. Use judgment when exercising.

****

Cold Therapy: A Shock to the System

You might not associate cold therapy with exercise, and very rightly so. But what if I told you that it's a vital component of my routine, one that has helped me immensely in the last few years? A few times a week, I like to expose my body to cold temperatures, either through the means of a cold shower or a cryo chamber. The shock to the system is invigorating in nature, it can reduce inflammation and increase the overall energy levels. Here are some of the benefits of cold therapy that I have experienced in the last few months(Espeland et al., n.d.).

- The experience of cold exposure feels like a jolt of electricity. But this jolt can prove to be quite beneficial for you. Cold therapy can awaken your senses, enhance the overall alertness, and increase the overall energy levels. It is nothing short of an incredible way to kick start your day.
- We know at this point in our discussion that inflammation is the body's natural response to injury or infection. But if you are suffering from chronic inflammation, this can prove to be quite detrimental for you. Cancer patients often experience chronic inflammation. Cold therapy, with its anti-inflammatory

effects, has the ability to reduce the overall inflammation and potentially limit cancer progression.

- Cold therapy can help reduce muscle soreness and enhance recovery. If you are engaging in intense exercises on a daily basis, cold therapy can feel like a natural ice bath for your body, one that can promote faster healing.

Now, if one can combine daily walking and rebounding, it can certainly prove to be a game-changer in their cancer journey. These three components of my exercise routine have provided me with a sense of physical and emotional well-being that helped me combat the side effects of cancer plus cancer treatments.

****

The Science behind Exercise and Cancer

So, why was I so persistent about my exercise routine, a question that you may ask.

Well, this was not something that was supported by speculation, rather, it has basis in science, and the evidence is super inspiring. Courtesy of the fact that we are living in 2023, the impact of exercise on cancer has been well-documented. It offers hope and tangible benefits to those who are trying their best to defeat cancer(Rajarajeswaran & Vishnupriya, 2009).

1. Cancer and its treatments can make you feel super fatigued, weak, and nauseous all at the same time. However, if you regularly exercise, you have a chance to feel pretty good about yourself. Exercise can help cut down common side effects, while also keeping your muscles strong, your weight in check, and your heart healthy. Multiple research studies back the fact that cancer patients who engage in exercise have reported improved physical functioning and a much improved quality of life.

2. Cancer is a disease that can prove to be super emotionally draining. For me, the simple acts of walking and rebounding became a source of happiness, they lifted my mood and eased the feelings of depression and anxiety. My confidence was back, and the exercise kind of sharpened my mind. Basically, it helped me cope with the stress. Research studies tell us that a few minutes of exercise can lead to substantial improvements in psychological well-being. Some of these improvements include reduced anxiety, increased self-esteem, and an improvement in the overall quality of life.

3. Our immune system is our first line of defense against cancer. Exercise is an immune system booster. Read two sentences together, and you can guess where we are going with this discussion. Exercise can strengthen our body's defenses, making it more resilient against infections and diseases. Research has already established that exercise can enhance immune function and reduce the risk of infections, something that is often a primary risk for cancer patients.

4. Inflammation is cancer's ally. But by staying active, you can counter inflammation too. It helps to control chronic inflammation, and in the process, makes it hard for cancer to thrive. Chronic inflammation and cancer progression have been linked together often. And because exercise has an anti-inflammatory effect, it can benefit those dealing with chronic inflammation immensely.

5. When I indulged in exercise, I found that I could better tolerate the side effects of treatments borne off chemotherapy and radiation. Research also backs what I found, and says that exercise can reduce the severity and impact of treatment-related side effects

6. Even today, for lucky survivors like me, exercise is like a protective shield. It reduces the risk of cancer relapse, and establishes a sense of security in my life. Science has established already that exercise is associated with a lower risk of cancer recurrence, so I have no worries in doing 20 minute walks and rebounding as much as I can!

****

Building an Exercise Program for Cancer Recovery

Now, if you are looking to build your own exercise program for accelerating and aiding your cancer recovery, here are some tips for you:

1. Please talk to your healthcare providers about your exercise plans, they can ensure that the plan aligns well with your unique circumstances.

2. If you were not active before your diagnosis, it is best to start slow. You can gradually build up your routine and avoid overexertion.

3. Safety is always going to be the number one priority. Please choose exercises, which will minimize the risk of injury. This holds true especially if you have had surgery or other cancer treatments previously.

4. Proper hydration is necessary when you exercise, especially when treatments like chemotherapy and radiation are already in place.

5. Lastly, it is very important to be realistic about your exercise goals. One must understand that their progress might be slower than others might, but it is perfectly ok!

****

As we saw it together in this chapter, exercise is more than just physical movement for patients suffering from cancer. Rather, it is an act of reclaiming your life. For me, it felt like a message to cancer: you are not the one who defines who I am. For me, exercise is now an essential tool on the path to recovery, an act that helps you regain physical and emotional well-being. We also saw how scientific evidence has illuminated the path, how it endorses the fact that exercise can enhance physical well-being, elevate mental health, reinforce the immune system, cut inflammation, improve treatment tolerance, and reduce the risk of cancer recurrence by a significant factor.

If you have to talk to your healthcare professional, do it. If you are going to do it yourself, do it. But please develop an exercise routine plan that you can easily follow, and you will see the results in no time.

Chapter 9: Mind Body Connection

Introduction

In my cancer journey, the interplay between my mind and body assumed a focal point, a focal point that was important to my transformative odyssey. Beyond the obvious challenges and medical complexities, I found myself in a position where mental well-being became a cornerstone of my recovery. True, I was still grappling with the initial shock of my diagnosis. But at the same time, it traversed the arduous path of treatment. Furthermore, I was able to confront the uncertainties that shrouded my future. I became fully aware of the massive impact that cultivating a positive mindset could have on my life.

In these lines, we will have a look at the significance of mental health in the face of cancer, we will realize how it can practically take center stage. These lines are not only a reminder of my physical battles, but also an exploration of the resilience, hope, and transformative power that was deeply embedded in the subtle nuances of the mind-body connection. Join me, as we unravel the strategies borne out of my conscious efforts to steer my thoughts toward healing. I tried my best to visualize a future that was free from the clutches of illness.

For me, these lines are not a personal narrative only. Rather it is a shared journey, a testament to the intricate dance between the conscious and the subconscious efforts. May my experiences serve as a guiding light and offer insights into the profound synergy between the mind and body in the realm of cancer recovery.

Believing that it is possible with supporting actions is power!

As simplistic as it sounds - the question drives the answer! I asked myself - "How am I going to help myself get rid of this disease and become completely healthy"?

Significance of Mental Well-being in Cancer Recovery

What exactly does mental well-being contribute to the cancer recovery trajectory? This is the main question that needs to be answered.

The question of the significance of mental well-being in cancer recovery quite delicately weaves into the fabric of my journey. Amid the labyrinth of treatment protocols and medical intricacies, it was all a quest for the answer to the question that I mentioned earlier.

To understand the importance of cancer recovery, we have to dive deep into the emotional contours of a cancer diagnosis. The initial shock becomes a forerunner to an emotional journey—a journey that is riddled with fear, uncertainty, and vulnerability. Think of it, not as an abstract concept, but as a tangible force, one that can influence the trajectory of healing massively.

One has to dissect the layers of emotional resonance that are embedded in the central question. The idea is to nurture a positive mindset. And for that to happen, one has to recognize that the battle against cancer is something beyond the physiological. It is all about building emotional resilience and understanding how mental fortitude can become a guiding light in shaping one's recovery process(Fernando, 2020).

My Mindful Approach to Thoughts

How are you thinking today?

This is the question that I used to ask myself a lot. I changed the way I was thinking about things, and by things, I mostly mean the cancer treatment protocols. Suddenly, I realized that I could influence my well-being. It was like steering a ship—one that I could guide in the right direction. I started practicing mindfulness every day.

Sounds a little complicated; I know.

But it is all about taking a few moments to be aware of your thoughts and enhance your focus on your mind. Have you ever realized how much our minds are like programmed computers? That is how marketers and advertisers make us buy things.

In a somewhat similar manner, I too decided to take charge of my thoughts. Now, I wanted my thoughts to be positive, filled with hope and healing. If you think a little deeply, it is like training your mind, it is all about making a conscious effort to shape your effort in a way that supports your health.

So how did I go about things? Well, I started spending about 15-20 minutes each day practicing mindfulness. This practice became the foundation for my healing. I learned that thoughts aren't just fleeting ideas—it is far from that. They are a powerful force that can shape our reality. Today's world is full of external influences. And that is where mindfulness can become anyone's fortress, it can protect your mental well-being amidst the chaos of cancer.

Sounds like a simple practice, yes?

But it made a massive difference in steering my thoughts toward health and positivity. In the face of adversity such as cancer, if one can not take control of their thoughts, choosing a path of healing becomes quite difficult.

****

Power of Visualization in Healing

Athletes often say that when they visualize themselves winning at certain sports, they feel more confident about winning. It was just like that for me as well, visualizing healing and being completely healthy became a potent tool in my arsenal against cancer.

Cancer is not going to go away, just because you are wishing it to go away. Rather, it's a mental rehearsal, a conscious effort to picture your body on the path to recovery. I would like you to imagine it as a vivid mental movie—just picture cancer cells diminishing and your overall well-being flourishing. It aligns with principles from mind-body medicine.

Please always remember that the mind is a powerful ally in the healing process. Visualization can tap into our mind's ability to shape our reality. It is as if one is creating a roadmap for the body to follow. Research studies have also supported this idea—visualizing positive outcomes can impact our physical well-being.

And this is how the transformative process began. For me, this practice became a daily ritual, there were at least a few moments in my day, where I used to close my eyes and envision my body healing.

There is something that must be stated clearly here. It's not about snubbing the challenges; rather it's about creating a mental space where healing is feasible, it is possible. Our mind can influence the body, and in this context, visualization is just like sending a positive message to every cell in our body.

Of course, visualization is a personal journey. However, the principles behind it are grounded in the idea that the mind and body are interconnected. The transformative influence of visualization can play a significant role in the intricate dance of healing from within.

****

Mindful Movement: Joyful Connection with the Body

In the rather depressing landscape of cancer, the application of practical techniques assumes massive importance, especially for patients who are struggling hard in terms of navigating this challenging journey. Cancer's emotional toll can be massive, absolutely crippling. One has to incorporate strategies that promote not only physical well-being but also provide the much-needed boost for mental resilience.

In this context, mindfulness practices are nothing short of invaluable tools. Tools that can provide amazing benefits for patients grappling with the uncertainties of cancer. Take the example of meditation here, a technique with a focus on the present moment. Meditation can provide enormous advantages, a refuge from the anxieties that often swirl in the minds of cancer patients. Deep breathing exercises can often bring a sense of calm amidst the storm of emotions in a cancer patient's life. By engaging in a simple act of becoming more aware of the breath, cancer patients can create a space for reflection and emotional healing.

It is all about finding little moments for physical and emotional relief. Here, practices like yoga, tai chi, exercise, walking, jogging or martial arts intertwine breath with movement and are of extreme interest, since they not only promote flexibility but also bring much-needed balance to one's life. If you can incorporate a structured routine into your life, you can regain a sense of control over your life amid the chaos of cancer treatment.

****

Scientific Insights into Mind-Body Connection

The research studies conducted thus far successfully illuminate the tangible impact of positive thoughts on a person's physical health. Neuroscientific studies tell us how our brains can respond to stress. This response influences immune function. Chronic stress, a common feature in cancer, can often lead to overproduction of cortisol. Cortisol is a hormone that can have a very negative impact on our body.

In such studies, the concept of neuroplasticity has been studied as well. Our brain can reorganize and form new neural connections, just tells you a lot about the adaptable nature of the brain, doesn't it? If you can keep a positive aura around yourself, chances are quite high that you will be able to find peace in your life, a lot sooner than you would expect(Chaoul et al., 2014).

****

Hormones, Stress, and Healing: Endocrine Perspectives

Let us talk a little bit more about hormones.

The endocrine system in our body is a complex network of glands and hormones. This system plays a massively important role in regulating our body's response to stress. Furthermore, it can accelerate the process of healing during cancer. As I mentioned earlier, chronic stress leads to the release of cortisol. It is a very important hormone that is produced by our adrenal glands. But while cortisol is essential for various bodily functions, too much cortisol can lead to detrimental effects on the human body, the most significant one in this discussion is perhaps, the suppression of the immune system.

It is at this point that our body is searching for ways in which it can counter the elevated levels of cortisol. This is where mindfulness techniques, for example, meditation and deep breathing can lead to an effective management of stress and cortisol levels. It becomes realistically more possible to create a supportive hormonal environment in which the recovery from cancer can proceed at a decent pace.

There might be individual variations in hormonal responses, doctors are very observant of that. And it is these variations that eventually allow for tailored interventions, one which can address specific needs. Eventually, it is these variations that give us clues about the development of integrative strategies.

****

Epigenetics: Lifestyle's Influence on Genetic Expression

First things first, what exactly is epigenetics?

Simply put, it is the study of changes in gene activity, but these changes do not involve alterations to the underlying DNA sequence(Hamilton, 2011).

Lifestyle choices, contemporary diet, exercise, and stress management all can exert massive influence on genetic expression. We have talked about the impact of diet at length previously, that is just one example of lifestyle's influence on genetic expression.

The key point to understand here is that the influence of epigenetics allows individuals to make informed choices, choices that could actively contribute to their well-being. Personalized lifestyle modifications are now a cornerstone in the comprehensive approach to cancer care, and subtle nuances are now being acknowledged in cancer treatment.

****

Social Support and Cognitive Behavioral Strategies

One cannot deny the importance of social support and cognitive-behavioral strategies at any point during cancer care. They often emerge as critical elements for emotional well-being. If you have a strong and impactful social network around you, it is going to provide you, not only practical assistance but can also serve as an emotional anchor. It is pertinent to mention here that your family, friends, and community connections can offer a sense of belonging and understanding unlike any other mechanism can. This sense of belonging can prove instrumental in alleviating the isolation associated with cancer diagnosis.

Researchers believe that cognitive-behavioral strategies can equip one with practical knowledge for combating mental and emotional challenges linked with cancer. These strategies are all about identifying and modifying negative thought patterns and then promoting adaptive mechanisms that could help you cope with challenges of all sorts. Here, one must not forget the concept of cognitive restructuring, an idea that empowers individuals to challenge and change harmful thought patterns, something that eventually contributes positively to life.

Support groups are amazing too, you know. Whether in-person or online, sports groups can always provide a much-needed sense of relief for individuals to share experiences, gain insights, and receive encouragement. It is a source of inspiration that any cancer patient can look to add at any point in their life. As you would realize it is all about approaching things from a holistic point of view!

****

Therefore, we reach the end of another chapter. However, hopefully, these lines will provide you with a comprehensive overview of the approach needed in cancer care. I am sure that you will agree with me that this approach involves a multifaceted integration of practical techniques as well as mindful movement, scientific insights, hormonal balance, epigenetic considerations, and robust social and cognitive support. It is all of these factors, which come into play together and contribute massively to one's overall wellbeing.

Chapter 10: Navigating the Challenges

The journey through cancer treatment is a complex and arduous road. It is often filled with unexpected challenges. From emotional turbulence to physical tolls, from financial strains to anxiety eating you all the time, each step in this journey is a unique hurdle. Overcoming these hurdles demands resilience, adaptability, and a robust support system. In the following lines, we will examine the setbacks and challenges faced during cancer treatment.

This is just not my story of hardships. Rather, it is something that individuals navigating cancer treatment often face. Furthermore, we will also look at the strategies you can employ to overcome these obstacles and offer encouragement for those facing similar trials.

Challenges

On the face of it, cancer treatment is more than a series of medical interventions. Instead, it's a transformative journey encompassing an individual's physical, emotional, and social dimensions. Patients and their loved ones navigate this intricate path as they encounter challenges. Sometimes, these challenges are beyond the realms of medical protocols. Understanding and addressing these challenges holistically is one of the most crucial aspects of providing comprehensive cancer care. Let's look at these challenges separately in the following lines.

1. Emotional Turbulence

Emotional impact is one of the most significant setbacks and challenges that a cancer patient can face. The impact of a cancer diagnosis is often very profound. It is far-reaching. Fear and anxiety are common responses to this overwhelming realization. And what is that realization, you may ask? Life has taken an unexpected turn. Coping with this emotional turmoil requires a multifaceted approach. Patients often seek mental health professionals as well as support groups and counseling services for navigating through intense emotions. But I found that the first thing that one must do is rely on the close circle of people who have been around you for an extended period. It could be family, it could be friends, or it could be a mixture of both. It is only after understanding the normalcy of such reactions and fostering an open dialogue about cancer treatment that one can mitigate the emotional challenges that are associated with cancer. You can also find solace in creative outlets such as therapy or journaling. Expressing emotions through various mediums is often found to be therapeutic. It helps to process complex feelings and find moments of clarity(McDaniel et al., 2021).

2. Treatment Side Effects

Then, there are the treatment side effects themselves. The physical toll of cancer treatments, while they are necessary for combating the disease, can be challenging to counter. Nausea, fatigue, and changes in physical appearance are not just physical challenges but also contribute massively to emotional distress. Strategies for managing treatment side effects often involve close collaboration between patients and healthcare providers. In this regard, nutritional counseling is of extreme importance. It can address challenges in appetite and weight. This ensures that the patients receive adequate nourishment despite the treatment-related challenges. Then, there are integrative therapies, for example, acupuncture or massage. These therapies can also alleviate some of the physical discomforts. Furthermore, open communication with the medical team is one of the most essential prerequisites for tailoring treatment plans and promptly addressing side effects. These approaches can then enhance the overall quality of life during cancer treatment by a significant factor.

3. Financial Strains

Nothing hits like a financial strain during the cancer treatment. The financial burden associated with cancer treatment is a very harsh reality for many folks. Navigating insurance, understanding copayments, and finding assistance programs are some of the most overwhelming feelings. To alleviate the financial strain, many folks have dedicated financial counselors. These counselors work with patients to explore available resources. Not only do they negotiate bills, but they also guide managing costs. Community organizations and nonprofits often offer financial assistance to cancer patients. If one can create awareness about these sources and foster partnerships between healthcare institutions and support organizations, the financial challenges faced by new patients undergoing cancer treatment can be eased significantly.

4. Physical Limitations

One also has to address the physical limitations of the process itself. This is a continuous adaptation process to physical limitations resulting from surgery, radiation, or chemotherapy. Physical therapy is considered to be pivotal and influential in helping patients regain mobility and independence. Beyond the clinical setting, embracing adaptive strategies and assistive devices is supportive in enhancing the day-to-day life of individuals facing physical challenges. Then, there are peer support groups where cancer patients can share their experiences and insights on adapting to physical challenges. This whole experience is often found to be very empowering. The peer support groups provide a sense of community and understanding. This reinforces the idea that life after a cancer diagnosis can still be fulfilling and meaningful. All that one has to do is find a friendly group to share your thoughts and challenges.

5. Uncertain Prognosis

Uncertain prognosis is a unique challenge. Countering it requires resilience and a shift in mindset. Many folks find that a balance between realistic optimism and living in the present moment is the key to countering uncertain prognosis. Palliative care focuses on enhancing the quality of life, and it has become an integral part of the treatment plan for cancer. It offers support and symptom management. If one can encourage open conversations between patients and their families and healthcare providers, treatments' potential outcomes and goals are well established. As a result of all this communication, a shared understanding is developed between all the members of this hierarchy. Advanced care planning, which includes discussions about end-of-life preferences, ensures that individuals retain control over their healthcare decisions. This provides them with a sense of agency in the face of uncertainty(Hui et al., 2019).

6. Social Isolation

One can also not ignore the social isolation that results from a combination of physical limitations, treatment schedules, and the stigma that is often associated with cancer. Combating social isolation is a step that requires creating a supportive network for patients. Friends and family are often considerably vital in maintaining these connections. Sometimes, it means adapting social activities to complete the patient's energy levels and needs. Community organizations and online support groups often offer avenues for social engagement. Integrating psychosocial support into the overall cancer care plan is a critical step that ensures that the patients and the assistant not only manage the physical aspects of the treatment but also navigate the complex social dynamics that may arise.

Strategies to Counter Challenges

Now, let us look at the strategies that can be employed to overcome these challenges.

1. Comprehensive Support Programs

Comprehensive support programs within cancer care institutions are pivotal in mitigating challenges. These programs often include a multidisciplinary team of healthcare professionals. These include oncologists, nurses, social workers, and mental health specialists. The idea is to ensure that patients receive medical care and holistic support that meets their needs.

Patient navigation services are often one's best bet for a dedicated professional guide; they guide patients through various aspects of their cancer journey. This approach can reduce the complexity of the healthcare system. These navigators help with appointment scheduling, financial assistance applications, and emotional support as a consistent point of contact throughout treatment. Now, that is a lot of help.

2. Integrative Therapies

Integrative therapies, which include acupuncture, yoga, and meditation, are increasingly becoming popular for their role in supporting cancer patients(Semeniuk et al., 2023). These approaches address both physical and emotional challenges. Of course, they are not substitutes for conventional medical treatments, but they complement the overall care plan by promoting relaxation, reducing stress, and improving overall well-being.

Then, incorporating alternative therapies, such as herbal supplements or dietary adjustments, is also intelligent. It is often done under the guidance of healthcare professionals. Cancer individuals find them beneficial in managing specific symptoms and enhancing their quality of life.

3. Empowerment Through Education

Education empowers patients to participate in their care; it helps them make informed decisions actively. Cancer education programs, workshops, and informational materials are often given secondary importance. But they can help patients understand their diagnosis, treatment options, and potential side effects. This knowledge equips individuals to communicate with their healthcare team; it fosters a sense of agency and involvement in decision-making.

Digital health platforms and online resources are also crucial in providing accessible and up-to-date information. Patient advocacy organizations often offer webinars and educational materials, serving as valuable sources of support and information for patients undergoing cancer treatment.

4. Advocacy for Policy Change

Addressing the financial challenges associated with cancer often requires systemic changes. Advocacy for local, regional, and national policy changes can improve insurance coverage, reduce out-of-pocket costs, and enhance access to affordable cancer care. Of course, this is something for the future, but a change in the policy would be a pleasant and welcome move that many cancer patients would appreciate.

Patient advocacy groups, alongside healthcare professionals, can engage with policymakers, thereby raising awareness about the financial burden faced by cancer patients. Through this advocacy, the broader community can contribute to a more supportive environment for cancer care patients.

5. Fostering Peer-Support Network

Peer support networks provide a source of encouragement built on shared experiences. If one can connect with individuals who have faced similar challenges, it can reduce feelings of isolation and offer practical insights into coping strategies.

Many cancer centers facilitate peer support programs or connect patients with survivorship groups.

Then, there are social media platforms, which are basically conduits for building virtual communities. Here, cancer patients can share their stories, seek advice, and support others in similar situations. Harnessing the power of peer support fosters a sense of belonging and resilience; it reinforces that individuals are not alone in their journey.

Encouragement for Readers Facing Similar Challenges

If you have been undergoing cancer treatment for some time, it's essential to recognize the strength within and around you. The journey may be demanding, but resilience, hope, and the capacity to adapt are potent backers. Let us look at some affirmations and encouragement for those facing similar challenges!

1. You Are Not Alone!

Reach out to your support network. This is massively important. Whether with friends, family, or support groups, sharing your journey is one of the most effective tools for sharing emotional burdens and strengthening your connections.

2. Embrace Your Strength

Acknowledge your inner strength. Every single moment, you have to keep reminding yourself of this. Every step, no matter how small, is a testament to your resilience. Hence, it becomes essential to celebrate your victories, no matter how incremental they may seem.

3. Advocate for Yourself

Be active in your care; do not depend on your medical team. Ask questions, seek second opinions, and voice your concerns. The opinions that you can provide are invaluable in shaping your treatment plan.

4. Celebrate Small Wins

Recognize and praise the small victories along the way. Whether completing a treatment cycle, handling a side effect, or finding moments of joy, these milestones matter.

5. Seek Professional Support

Mental health is an integral part of your well-being. Don't waver to seek support from mental health specialists specializing in oncology. They can provide coping methods and a safe space to express your emotions.

6. Explore Integrative Therapies

Integrative therapies can improve your overall well-being when aligned with your medical treatment. Explore mindfulness, yoga, or acupuncture opportunities to find what resonates with you.

7. Be Patient with Yourself

Understand that this journey is not linear, and recovery is a process. Be patient with yourself, accepting that healing takes time.

8. Engage in Advocacy

If you feel compelled, consider engaging in advocacy efforts. Your say can contribute to systemic modifications that benefit you and future cancer patients.

9. Connect with Peers

Peer help can be a lifeline. Join with others who have faced similar challenges. Sharing experiences and understanding can provide a sense of understanding and camaraderie.

10. Celebrate Life

Amidst the challenges, find instants to commemorate life. Whether it's enjoying a hobby, spending time with loved ones, or savoring simple joys, these moments add profoundness to your journey.

So there you are. Now, we are aware of some of the challenges that we might face during our cancer treatment journey and how we can navigate through them. It is just a glimpse, though; you can achieve much more than you think!

Chapter 11: Importance of Hope

They say hope is one of the greatest allies supporting quality of life.

For cancer patients, it becomes doubly true.

For me, I cannot even think of a day where I was not mentally focusing on getting through this terrible ordeal. I saw hope as a significant tool of empowerment. It was an element in which I saw hope as a primary empowerment tool.

Hope, the will to live, all the time thinking about a better time, all these thoughts were essentially one in nature. For cancer patients, hope is often read and interpreted as remission. Truth to be told, it is perhaps the best definition. But, the central idea is to not only avert death but follow a path through medical treatment and support that can have a long-lasting impact on our lives. From hoping for treatments that can cure or palliate the disease to resuming our journey in everyday life, a cancer patient goes through a lot of phases - I sure did! One principle that I still adhere to daily is practicing gratitude, hope and never giving up!

****

If I were to refer to classical literature for the first time in this book, the Oxford dictionary's definition of hope inspired me. Oxford dictionary says that hope can entertain the expectations of something you are desirous of. In other words, hope embodies an emotional component beyond expectation. It is an integral part of the human experience. There is no second thought about that in my mind. Plants and trees are often bent towards the sun's warmth. Don't you think it is comparable to a person's hope for improved survival?

****

Scribbling these lines as an author is less critical than telling you my tale as a fellow traveler on this winding road of life. My story is a testament to the incredible power of hope and an illuminating path that my fellow cancer patients could walk on.

The word cancer itself, let a lone stage four cancer can cause a very heavy shadow on one's life. It comes with a darkness that seems impossible to penetrate - but with faith, hope and a plan it is possible. I am literally living proof!

But even within this darkness was a flicker of light, a light that I called hope. It was a light that, against all the odds, guided me through the toughest of times. At this point in this journey, you're well aware that my journey began with a cancer diagnosis that echoed through the corridors of my life. It reverberated with fear, uncertainty, and questions I had no answers to, at least back then. Cancer was a terrible phase that I never thought I would encounter or face in my life - let alone Stage IV cancer! But as I started nurturing hope, I realized I could weather the most brutal storms of my life with the right attitude.

Courage is knowing when to be afraid. Plato believed in that. After fighting cancer for such a long time, I agree with Plato. I know many people who have faced serious illnesses and yet they managed to not be overwhelmed by the magnitude of the disorders. Yes, they fell ill and thought about giving up, but the part to focus upon is that they never gave up. The body suffers, yes. But if your spirit remains strong, you can overcome any worldly challenge, provided it is not beyond your physical and mental capacity. Throughout my healing journey I focused on the positive and guided my mind to remember the good that awaited me!

****

Life threatening illnesses are a reminder that we are not immortal. But, those who respond creatively to a life-threatening illness see this moment as a wake-up call. For them, it comes as a reminder of how short the time is and how precious life is. So, in that moment of uncertainty, they do what matters the most. Rather than succumbing to the fear, they try to experience life and life's joys. They let the people around them know how much you love and appreciate them. For me, it became a simple matter of just dropping useless commitments, and a matter of trivializing the trivial. I started to drop useless commitments and eliminate relationships that were troubling and not worth my time. I started to say no to what did not serve me and made myself a priority - my life literally depended on it!

You will hear many stories of courageous people who became ill or faced other crises. And yet, one thing that you will read about these people is that they consider themselves very fortunate. In the face of a dismal disorder or disease, they can take stock of their resources and find strength and love. My fellow readers, this is something that I would also urge you to do as well.

****

Does it matter which stage your cancer is?

This is an important question. Of course, if someone is facing a short-term disorder that can be cured or *at least* tackled carefully using existing medicine and treatment protocols, then yes, the intensity of hope in that particular individual is going to be high. But if someone is suffering from a long-term disease, finding hope becomes even more critical. Survivors are well advised to hope for the best but prepare for the worst.

For me, being prepared for the worst part never worked well. There was always a part of me that wanted to live with hope for a cure, remission, or stable cancer without suffering and a treatment that would help me enjoy a high quality of life with my loved ones for as long as possible.

****

But here is something interesting. You can begin to lose hope if you are experiencing a loss of empathy and compassion. If you begin to withdraw yourself from reality, from your friends and family, and even from the medical support team, as is the case in some cancer patients, you might begin to experience psychologically depressing or destructive medical or social processes. For you, life will suddenly seem like a disappointing and unsatisfactory experience. While cancer is such a disorder that rightly makes one feel that way, one has to get out of this trap and stop it. This destructive pattern can have significant psychological implications. It indicates a process of utter despair.

So, the one thing that I started doing was I started to feel embedded in a network of caring at the time of serious illness. My will to live was not the denial of death; instead, it came as an intensification of life experience. And this can only come with the realization of how finite life truly is.

Given my diagnosis and current state - I consider myself extremely fortunate! Not only because I have and am navigating stage IV cancer, but because it has given me an immense appreciation for life!

As it is sometimes said - one does not appreciate things until they are gone! Well, I have faced the possibility of death and now have an immense appreciation for life!

In regards to treatment, for those of you who want to put a lot of faith in modern medical therapy or research literature, even the health professionals believe that a combination of medical therapy with the adoption of healthy lifestyles and supportive care offers a lot of improvement.

But all of this improvement is in vain if the patient is not willing to fight for themselves. It is a combination of all the things, you know, a comprehensive care plan that can address a wide range of needs for the cancer patient.

****

It is easier said than done. I perfectly understand this.

If you're diagnosed with cancer, chances are likely that you will fail to maintain a positive attitude for the weeks to follow. Would you mind confronting many obstacles? And of course, some of these are quite visible because of the side effects of the illness and the treatment. But then there are feelings of fear, anger, depression, and loneliness that no one talks about a lot these days. This is quite surprising because you would assume that the impact of these feelings on one's journey is such that they should be given priority and primary importance. But, in most hospitals, the focus is on chemotherapy, giving IV medicines, and ensuring the patient eats three meals. Some patients are happy with that, but the majority are not.

So, how to make sure that your lively, buoyant personality is not tarnished too much by cancer and feelings? One way of doing this is to maintain and set reasonable and achievable goals. How can you do this? Well, you are not going to be up and about, going to the parties when you are going through chemotherapy or associated treatments. That is not going to be the case.

****

But, you can form a social circle or a company around you that genuinely empathizes, cares about you, and can actually care about you and relate to what you are feeling. Cancer communities are excellent, but most of the time these communities lack the essential elements that the community should have. You have to put a lot of energy into activities that will satisfy you. And more often than not, the best way to perform these activities is to do them in a community or group formed by people like you.

****

Hope is something not everyone understands. You know, usually, we hope for something that we know. In other words, the variable is known. For example, you might hope that your team wins the World Series or Super Bowl..

But what is the future for cancer patients? Why should they keep hoping for something unknown to them? What kind of feeling do they need in their system to keep them alive to endure terrible treatments, and what are the side effects?

Well, the hope in this case is supported by the positive attitude of the medical team, but it can also be very fragile. Anything that demoralizes a person can negate the feeling of hope. Hence, if failure occurs, you're likely to experience a difference in accepting or denying the next set of treatments. Usually, the feeling of hope and will to live will vary daily, and depends on the physical status, psychological outlook, and the treatment success or failure. Depression or isolation in this context is significant.

But, having said all of that, hope is to be kept alive to live, and constantly live in gratitude for what we do have! Gratitude for being able to make choices about our treatment and help ourselves through lifestyle and diet changes. Otherwise, what are you looking at? What is the alternative? A feeling of despair, right? Well, hope is often a shared feeling with one's team of family and friends. But I will tell you this: if you can find the resolution to live and fight for another day, another month, another year, it is all about finding another opportunity to respond to cancer therapy and to live.

In the following lines, I share some quotes that will help you find the much-needed inspiration to tackle cancer:

"My life is different now, but it's still good."

— *Max Nickless, anaplastic thyroid cancer survivor*

"Don't give up. This is only temporary."

— *Ilyasha Hosea, breast cancer survivor*

"Some of life's sourest lemons make the best lemonade."

— *Ciara Toth, acute lymphoblastic leukemia survivor*

"Each of us has greater strength because of the other."

— *Ben Sanders, melanoma and prostate cancer survivor*

"Life can still be beautiful after cancer."

— *Alexa Jett, papillary thyroid cancer survivor*

"I still have some dark days. But now, I also have hope and optimism."

— *Elpida Argenziano, breast cancer survivor*

"Side effects are a small price to pay for my life."

— *Peggy Port, ovarian cancer survivor*

"All I want to do is live well and love deeply."

— *Nicole Body, sarcoma survivor*

"I choose to get busy living."

— *Constance Blanchard, glioblastoma survivor*

"Every single bad day is better than no day at all."

— *Deanna Wehrung, cervical cancer survivor*

"I have much to be happy about just because I'm a survivor."

— *Vanessa Sanders, breast cancer survivor*

Remember - you only have one life; so fight for it and live it!

****

Chapter 12: A Journey Beyond Cancer

Living My Best Life

While it does sound a little extraordinary, living my best life has become an extraordinary reality. Now, I'm surpassing anything that I could have imagined, especially during the darkest days of my cancer battle. This profound shift in my health and well-being is nothing short of a miracle. It is a testament to the resilience of the human spirit, something I keep encouraging you to read more about.

The journey into uncharted territory has transformed every aspect of my existence. Today, I wake up each day with renewed purpose and gratitude. I savor the simple joys that were once overshadowed by this specter of cancer. From tasting a nutrient-rich meal to the warmth of the morning sun, my life has taken on a vibrant hue. Colors that were once muted are now back in my life. This newfound energy courses through my veins as a constant reminder of the miraculous metamorphosis I've undergone. Every step that I take, every breath that I draw resonates with the vitality that cancer was stealing from me.

My life is a celebration; it is a celebration and an ode to the body's incredible capacity to heal and regenerate. A journey beyond cancer is not a triumph over a singular disease. Instead, it's a profound affirmation of the boundless possibilities that await us when we embrace life with open arms. In the following lines, I will unfold the layers of this transformation for you; I will reveal strategies, insights, and daily practices that have propelled me into the best of my life.

Scans Showing Cancer Arrest

Each set of scans that furnished good news felt like a breath of fresh air to me. Every scan was a profound story of cancer arrest. We were having these scans every three months, and I sensed that something was healing about the medical snapshots themselves. They were a powerful narrative of my resilience and triumph. Cancer, which was once rampant in my body, was now frozen. It was a visual representation of the effectiveness of the protocol. To others, they might appear as black-and-white representations. But for me, they were a testimony to the success of my protocol and the therapeutic measures that I had adopted. I must tell you something: the feeling of a sustained cessation is unreal!

The Protocol: My Ticket to a New Life

I have discussed my protocol with you at length already. I feel like revising its fundamentals once more here. The protocol was meticulously crafted and adhered to. It served as my compass, guiding me through uncharted territories of health. When I say that it's not just a regimen; it's my ticket to a new life, I am not half exaggerating. My protocol was built on nutrition, exercise, and a mindset overhaul; no wonder it became integral to my daily existence. I implore you to adopt this roadmap to steer you towards a sustainable well-being. The protocol was instrumental in rewriting my health narrative, making this protocol not just a regimen but a profound catalyst for transformation.

My Routine

My daily routine is a testament to the fact that life can change if you want to live. The transformative power of intentional living can be pretty astonishing. From the moment I wake up to the time I lay my head down, every action in my life now is a conscious step towards health, resilience, and life beyond cancer.

When the sun shines, I engage in mindfulness and meditation. Gratitude is very close to my heart now. Being grateful for the second opportunity in life sets the tone for the day ahead. It is pertinent to mention that these practices are not mere rituals for me. Instead, they're the foundation of my mental will, creating a space where positivity flourishes.

Breakfast time - well for me late lunch. My plate is usually filled with nutrient-rich, plant-based feast foods - spinach and kale based salads. My body is flooded with antioxidants, vitamins, and minerals. Each bite of my breakfast, actually lunch, is a deliberate choice to nourish my body's cellular environment, fostering an environment in which health can thrive. Then came the time for exercise, now I am able to walk or exercise while still fasting which is what I do! Exercise, as you all know, is essential. But in the last few years, it has become something non-negotiable. From taking a brisk walk to complementing it with stretching or resistance training, now I have dedicated time for moving my body. It's not all about physical fitness, either.

My obsession is keeping my body strong and ready for life's challenges. It's time for midday. Moment of mindfulness. And amid daily demands, I take a breath. A deep breath is vital. It bridges one to the present moment. It offers a respite from the chaos that cancer can often unleash. Mindfulness isn't a luxury; it is necessary to maintain balance in the whirlwind of life.

Then comes an after lunch healthy snack sometimes. A colorful array of selected fruits, vegetables, and nuts grace my plate. You might think of this diet as a somewhat restrictive diet. That is not the case (see Appendix for food list). Conscious choice for providing my body with the whole goodness it craves. Dense meals become a source of vitality for me. The afternoon is all about reflection, not dwelling on the past. Instead, it is a mindful acknowledgment of the present. Reflection often helps us assess energy, emotions, and other feelings, which can be adjusted accordingly. Afternoon is a practice in self-awareness and adaptability for me. The evening is here. It brings a sense of accomplishment. The day is filled with mindful choices.

What about the night? I make sure to drink my low calorie high quality organic celery juice. Also, typically I am not hungry at night. However, if I happen to be hungry at night, I will snack on some quality nuts. Fortunately for me, I am usually not hungry and do not indulge in excesses anymore. The intentional approach to life activities that keep me healthy has paid off well for me.

Keep in mind, I eat and drink juice within a maximum 8hr window daily - except on my 2 day weekly fast with IV Vitamin C when I only drink water and take my supplements!

****

Next, night falls upon the day and sleep comes. Sleep, sleep. Yep, sleep, I will. But I must tell you that sleep is not just rest. Instead, it is a crucial component of my well-being. I feel distraught if I do not have a good night's sleep. Having a good night's sleep is highly non-negotiable. Sleep hours, for me, are hours of rejuvenation. During this time, my body undergoes repairs and prepares me for the challenges of the new day. It's not a set of rigid rules, though. Instead, it's more dynamic and adaptable to the ebb and flow of life. Each element is a brush stroke on the canvas of a life I am living well. It's a conscious choice; it's a commitment to thriving, not just surviving.

Words of Encouragement

Fighting cancer is a formidable challenge. Demands resilience. An unwavering spirit is essential to fighting cancer. You have gone through the twists and turns of my life. You might have noticed that it is essential to recognize your steps and hail them as triumphs themselves. In the face of adversity, you must find strength to persevere.

It starts by acknowledging that setbacks are an inevitable part of the journey. Of course, there may be frustration, disappointment, and even despair. All of these emotions are valid, though. They are natural responses to the challenges we encounter. Cancer is a big challenge. But please understand one thing and keep it in your mind forever. Setbacks are synonymous with anything but failure. One can gain a compelling perspective. Each obstacle becomes an opportunity to learn, adapt, and emerge triumphant; and perspective is powerful. It is like transforming challenges into opportunities. One must embrace the power of a positive mindset. The road can be challenging. But each obstacle must be viewed as a temporary hurdle. It should not be an insurmountable wall. It has to shift from the typical journey to the beauty of the present moment.

As I mentioned, having a support system, whether friends, family, or community, is essential. Your experiences and learning about the subtle nuances of the cancer journey can help you draw strength from collective wisdom. Here, we are focused more on embracing a holistic approach to well-being, not just dependent on medical innovations but also on lifestyle choices that nurture our body, mind, and spirit. It is not about avoiding challenges; instead, it is about bouncing back from them. One can cultivate resilience by fostering adaptability. It helps one maintain a sense of purpose. It also helps one stay connected with the inner wellspring of strength. Life becomes quite pleasant if one can understand the resilience that grows with each trial faced and overcome.

Cancer is an overreaching battle. Hence, one must be very realistic and celebrate small victories. From completing a treatment cycle to managing symptoms effectively, from finding joy in a moment of reprieve, short wins are the threads that can weave the tapestry of your resilience. One has to acknowledge and savor the actual markers of your journey. And if your cancer journey has a lot of markers like these, indeed, you will find more strength every day.

So, what do you do on your most challenging days? It's a question that must have gone through your mind already. Well, let me answer it here now that we have discussed all the possible ways to counter cancer. You will have some tough days, I won't lie to you. The toll of the journey can feel quite overwhelming. One must give yourself some grace. It's okay to feel this weight of emotions. Acknowledging fear is not a bad thing. Being angry about something tormenting you constantly is not an issue. It is OK to feel sad sometimes. But I want you to remember that these emotions do not define you. You're a warrior by getting into uncharted territories with courage and grit. So, when overcoming challenges, aligning yourself to rest, meditating, and returning to the battle with renewed vigor is justified. Extending the same compassion to yourself that you would do to a dear friend is not only nice, but needed! Recognizing the normality of your challenge is quite important. It helps you understand what you are facing; it helps you honor the courage that it takes to beat a monstrous disease like cancer.

Healing is a multifaceted journey, and it's pretty essential. Every step of it is a victory. There will come a time when you will be looking beyond cancer. The battle with cancer is an interpretation of the narrative, yes. But it will never define your entire story. One has to look beyond the confines of the diagnosis. Only then can you envision a future filled with moments of joy, fulfillment, and purpose! Also, one has to allow their journey to shape them. Your personality must be shaped well enough. Oh, and always remember, encouragement is not just a sentiment. *It's a beacon of light that will illuminate your path in healing and life beyond cancer!*

Chapter 13: Ending on a High Note

Farewell and Reflections: Navigating the Cancer Challenge

Goodbyes are always the hardest, I am most disappointed that we must wrap up things now.

But this isn't a casual *thank you for reading my narrative* kind of conclusion.

I would rather you reflect on the myriad of challenges that paint the canvas of the cancer challenge.

From the initial shock of diagnosis to the relentless pursuit of healing, it is a tapestry of resilience, hope, setbacks, and triumphs. By triumph, I, of course, refer to the promise of a life beyond cancer.

From Setbacks to Triumphs: Unveiling the Tapestry of Resilience

When I look back, my journey through cancer, at least for me, resembles a profound odyssey. Every step that I took held the weight of both a challenge and a revelation. It was a roller coaster of emotions. My resilience was tested in the crucibles of adversity. Much credit to my unwavering spirit that refused to be diminished by the shadows of uncertainty.

All these tests have come together to form the fabric of my rather unique story.

Setbacks are an inevitable part of a journey. They play a very pivotal role in shaping narratives. From the moments of despair, we find courage. Trials that often seem insurmountable demand courage be summoned. Only then is it possible to face these obstacles head-on. And every time you summon a bit of courage, you contribute something to the rich tapestry of your experience. And that is where it becomes very important to acknowledge setbacks not as roadblocks but as stepping stones. They will guide you towards growth and newfound strength.

The strategies that I used to overcome obstacles were not just practical measures. Rather, they were a profound expression of resilience. The support systems woven into the journey, be it the company of loved ones, the collective support of the community, or the holistic approach to well-being, all contributed massively to fortifying my spirit to fight cancer. I have talked at length about the protocol. The value of the protocol lies in its proper implementation. And to help me implement the protocol, I will always be grateful to my closest friends and family. They helped me have a positive mindset. The transformative power of a positive mindset was instrumental in creating a road map to healing and proved to be instrumental in navigating the most challenging terrains.

Resilience became the heartbeat of this journey. It was my companion that grew stronger with every trial I faced. The ability to bounce back, find light in the darkest corners, and emerge from adversity to transform the narrative from mere survival to a celebration of the human spirit's indefatigable strength is a story that I will always cherish.

The Holistic Journey: Celebrating Small Victories & Embracing Hope

In the grand narrative of battling cancer, the importance of celebrating small victories cannot be overstated. From completing a treatment cycle to managing symptoms effectively, from finding joy in the simplest pleasures, which will then become milestones that illuminated the pathway forward, each trying became a testament to the resilience within my body.

I must also talk about hope here. A guiding light that illuminates the darkest corners when you're on the journey to defeating cancer. From the advances of medical science to the support of loved ones, from the unwavering belief in the resilience of the human spirit to implementing your protocol daily, you will find that hope is always there. It will serve as the compass that points you toward a brighter future. A future that is brimming with possibilities.

Most of the cancer patients often try to find solace. It is usually missing, and that is because they isolate themselves. Now, if you can find solace in connection, you have already conquered 40 to 50% of the battle. Shared experiences, empathy, exchange, and understanding drawn from others who have been through similar experiences become a source of profound comfort for everyone. An interconnectedness does exist in human experiences. This interconnectedness creates a sanctuary where understanding, support, and shared wisdom thrive.

Here, I must also talk about the value of self-compassion in the pursuit of healing. As you might have guessed, I relied on it a lot. I have realized that in the last few years, I have gotten very good at acknowledging the journey's enormity and extending kindness to others. It is an act of profound healing! My fellow campaigners for you, I want you to remember that patience with the process is one of the most important ingredients in this journey. Not only does it demand the acceptance of the journey's complexities, but it also requires one to honor the courage within pillars of self-compassion.

I was once a warrior in the throes of cancer.

Today, as you read my story, you must agree that it feels more like a testament to the transformative power of resilience and the will to survive and thrive. My ongoing health and wellness showcase not only the arrest of cancer but a renaissance of vitality. Stability coupled with regression is nothing but tangible proof of the efficacy of my protocol. You will have your doubts, and rightly so. I don't expect you to put all your faith in my protocol. Human nature is a rather curious phenomenon; it is not in our nature to trust everything we hear and read. However, I advise you to put your faith in my protocol and let scans dictate your steps. It worked better for me than most traditional stand alone treatments!

This narrative describing the depths of despair to the pinnacle of triumph, a testament to the extraordinary resilience inherent in the human spirit, has now reached a concluding point. The transformative journey emphasizes the importance of adopting a holistic approach to health. This approach is all about the fusion of conventional and complementary strategies, a harmonious balance between mind and body.

May my narrative serve as a beacon, guiding you through the labyrinth of uncertainty.

May it encourage you to believe unwaveringly in your innate capacity for healing.

I wish you a life filled with hope, purpose, and the boundless potential for healing beyond measure!

****

Food List

Key is Cruciferous Organic Plant Based

Avocados	Berries	Lemons	Limes
Arugula	Asparagus	Bell Peppers	Bok Choy
Broccoli	Brussel Sprouts	Cabbage	Cauliflower
Celery	Cucumbers	Eggplant	Garlic
Green Beans	Kale	Lettuce	Romaine
Mushrooms	Onions	Spinach	Squash
Tomatoes	Turnips	Zucchini	Salmon
Tuna	Sardines	Trout	Chicken
Turkey	Flaxseed Oil	MCT Oil	Guacamole
Salsa	Sauerkraut	Pickles	Almonds
Brazil Nuts	Hazelnuts	Walnuts	Macadamias
Olives	Seaweed	Broccoli Sprouts	

Wild Caught Fish   Organic Chicken

Organic Celery Juice and plenty of water!

Note - my main daily meal(s) was a *plant based salad*! The base was spinach, kale, and added different lettuce types to spruce it up.

References

1. Abdelaziz, A., & Vaishampayan, U. (2017). Cabozantinib for the treatment of kidney cancer. *Expert Review of Anticancer Therapy*, *17*(7), 577–584. https://doi.org/10.1080/14737140.2017.1344553

2. Adair, T. H., & Montani, J.-P. (2010). Overview of Angiogenesis. In *Angiogenesis*. Morgan & Claypool Life Sciences. https://www.ncbi.nlm.nih.gov/books/NBK53238/

3. Adekola, K., Rosen, S. T., & Shanmugam, M. (2012). Glucose transporters in cancer metabolism. *Current Opinion in Oncology*, *24*(6), 650–654. https://doi.org/10.1097/CCO.0b013e328356da72

4. Ağagündüz, D., Şahin, T. Ö., Yılmaz, B., Ekenci, K. D., Duyar Özer, Ş., & Capasso, R. (2022). Cruciferous Vegetables and Their Bioactive Metabolites: From Prevention to Novel Therapies of Colorectal Cancer. *Evidence-Based Complementary and Alternative Medicine : eCAM*, *2022*, 1534083. https://doi.org/10.1155/2022/1534083

5. Agrawal, S., Vamadevan, P., Mazibuko, N., Bannister, R., Swery, R., Wilson, S., & Edwards, S. (2019). A New Method for Ethical and Efficient Evidence Generation for Off-Label Medication Use in Oncology (A Case Study in Glioblastoma). *Frontiers in Pharmacology*, *10*, 681. https://doi.org/10.3389/fphar.2019.00681

6. Ahmed, K., Shaw, H. V., Koval, A., & Katanaev, V. L. (2016). A Second WNT for Old Drugs: Drug Repositioning against WNT-Dependent Cancers. *Cancers*, *8*(7), 66. https://doi.org/10.3390/cancers8070066

7. Amjad, M. T., Chidharla, A., & Kasi, A. (2023). Cancer Chemotherapy. In *StatPearls*. StatPearls Publishing. http://www.ncbi.nlm.nih.gov/books/NBK564367/

8. Bhutia, S. K., Mukhopadhyay, S., Sinha, N., Das, D. N., Panda, P. K., Patra, S. K., Maiti, T. K., Mandal, M., Dent, P., Wang, X.-Y., Das, S. K., Sarkar, D., & Fisher, P. B.

(2013). Autophagy: Cancer's Friend or Foe? *Advances in Cancer Research*, *118*, 61–95. https://doi.org/10.1016/B978-0-12-407173-5.00003-0

9. Brand, D. A. (2019). The Stage IV Shuffle: Elusiveness of Straight Talk About Advanced Cancer. *Journal of General Internal Medicine*, *34*(11), 2637–2642. https://doi.org/10.1007/s11606-019-05158-5

10. Cao, Y., Nishihara, R., Wu, K., Wang, M., Ogino, S., Willett, W. C., Spiegelman, D., Fuchs, C. S., Giovannucci, E. L., & Chan, A. T. (2016). Population-wide Impact of Long-term Use of Aspirin and the Risk for Cancer. *JAMA Oncology*, *2*(6), 762–769. https://doi.org/10.1001/jamaoncol.2015.6396

11. Chaoul, A., Milbury, K., Sood, A. K., Prinsloo, S., & Cohen, L. (2014). Mind-Body Practices in Cancer Care. *Current Oncology Reports*, *16*(12), 417. https://doi.org/10.1007/s11912-014-0417-x

12. Chen, G.-Q., Benthani, F. A., Wu, J., Liang, D., Bian, Z.-X., & Jiang, X. (2020). Artemisinin compounds sensitize cancer cells to ferroptosis by regulating iron homeostasis. *Cell Death and Differentiation*, *27*(1), 242–254. https://doi.org/10.1038/s41418-019-0352-3

13. Curigliano, G., & Criscitiello, C. (2014). Successes and limitations of targeted cancer therapy in breast cancer. *Progress in Tumor Research*, *41*, 15–35. https://doi.org/10.1159/000355896

14. D'Eliseo, D., & Velotti, F. (2016). Omega-3 Fatty Acids and Cancer Cell Cytotoxicity: Implications for Multi-Targeted Cancer Therapy. *Journal of Clinical Medicine*, *5*(2), 15. https://doi.org/10.3390/jcm5020015

15. Dhawan, D. K., & Chadha, V. D. (2010). Zinc: A promising agent in dietary chemoprevention of cancer. *The Indian Journal of Medical Research*, *132*(6), 676–682.

16. Dogra, N., Kumar, A., & Mukhopadhyay, T. (2018). Fenbendazole acts as a moderate microtubule destabilizing agent and causes cancer cell death by modulating multiple

cellular pathways. *Scientific Reports*, *8*, 11926. https://doi.org/10.1038/s41598-018-30158-6

17. Downer, S., Berkowitz, S. A., Harlan, T. S., Olstad, D. L., & Mozaffarian, D. (2020). Food is medicine: Actions to integrate food and nutrition into healthcare. *The BMJ*, *369*, m2482. https://doi.org/10.1136/bmj.m2482

18. Espeland, D., de Weerd, L., & Mercer, J. B. (n.d.). Health effects of voluntary exposure to cold water – a continuing subject of debate. *International Journal of Circumpolar Health*, *81*(1), 2111789. https://doi.org/10.1080/22423982.2022.2111789

19. Faden, A. A. (2016). The potential role of microbes in oncogenesis with particular emphasis on oral cancer. *Saudi Medical Journal*, *37*(6), 607–612. https://doi.org/10.15537/smj.2016.6.14048

20. Fernández-Lázaro, D., Mielgo-Ayuso, J., Córdova Martínez, A., & Seco-Calvo, J. (2020). Iron and Physical Activity: Bioavailability Enhancers, Properties of Black Pepper (Bioperine®) and Potential Applications. *Nutrients*, *12*(6), 1886. https://doi.org/10.3390/nu12061886

21. Fernando, A. (2020). Mental Health and Cancer: Why It Is Time to Innovate and Integrate—A Call to Action. *European Urology Focus*, *6*(6), 1165–1167. https://doi.org/10.1016/j.euf.2020.06.025

22. Ghaffari, H., Atashzar, M. R., & Abdollahi, H. (2020). Molecular imaging in tracking cancer stem cells: A review. *Medical Journal of the Islamic Republic of Iran*, *34*, 90. https://doi.org/10.34171/mjiri.34.90

23. Gilbert, R. W., Kim, J. H., & Posner, J. B. (1978). Epidural spinal cord compression from metastatic tumor: Diagnosis and treatment. *Annals of Neurology*, *3*(1), 40–51. https://doi.org/10.1002/ana.410030107

24. Giordano, A., & Tommonaro, G. (2019). Curcumin and Cancer. *Nutrients*, *11*(10), 2376. https://doi.org/10.3390/nu11102376

25. Goel, P., & Gerriets, V. (2023). Chloroquine. In *StatPearls*. StatPearls Publishing. http://www.ncbi.nlm.nih.gov/books/NBK551512/

26. González, M. J., Miranda-Massari, J. R., Mora, E. M., Guzmán, A., Riordan, N. H., Riordan, H. D., Casciari, J. J., Jackson, J. A., & Román-Franco, A. (2005). Orthomolecular Oncology Review: Ascorbic Acid and Cancer 25 Years Later. *Integrative Cancer Therapies*, *4*(1), 32–44. https://doi.org/10.1177/1534735404273861

27. Gyamfi, J., Kim, J., & Choi, J. (2022). Cancer as a Metabolic Disorder. *International Journal of Molecular Sciences*, *23*(3), 1155. https://doi.org/10.3390/ijms23031155

28. Gyanani, V., Haley, J. C., & Goswami, R. (2021). Challenges of Current Anticancer Treatment Approaches with Focus on Liposomal Drug Delivery Systems. *Pharmaceuticals*, *14*(9), 835. https://doi.org/10.3390/ph14090835

29. Haines, I., Elliott, P., & Stanley, R. (2011). Rituximab-containing therapy for chronic lymphocytic leukaemia-Authors reply. *Lancet*, *377*, 205; author reply 206. https://doi.org/10.1016/S0140-6736(11)60042-1

30. Hamilton, J. P. (2011). Epigenetics: Principles and Practice. *Digestive Diseases (Basel, Switzerland)*, *29*(2), 130–135. https://doi.org/10.1159/000323874

31. Higdon, J. V., Delage, B., Williams, D. E., & Dashwood, R. H. (2007). Cruciferous Vegetables and Human Cancer Risk: Epidemiologic Evidence and Mechanistic Basis. *Pharmacological Research : The Official Journal of the Italian Pharmacological Society*, *55*(3), 224–236. https://doi.org/10.1016/j.phrs.2007.01.009

32. Hormone replacement therapy and cancer. (2001). *Gynecological Endocrinology: The Official Journal of the International Society of Gynecological Endocrinology*, *15*(6), 453–465.

33. Huang, Y.-T., Lin, Y.-W., Chiu, H.-M., & Chiang, B.-H. (2016). Curcumin Induces Apoptosis of Colorectal Cancer Stem Cells by Coupling with CD44 Marker. *Journal of Agricultural and Food Chemistry*, *64*(11), 2247–2253.

https://doi.org/10.1021/acs.jafc.5b05649

34. Hui, D., Maxwell, J. P., & Paiva, C. E. (2019). Dealing with Prognostic Uncertainty: The Role of Prognostic Models and Websites for Patients with Advanced Cancer. *Current Opinion in Supportive and Palliative Care, 13*(4), 360–368. https://doi.org/10.1097/SPC.0000000000000459

35. Ipilimumab (Yervoy) in combination with nivolumab (Opdivo) for the first-line treatment of advanced renal cell cancer: Ipilimumab (Yervoy) and nivolumab (Opdivo) for the first-line treatment of advanced renal cell cancer with an intermediate prognosis. (2019). In *InformedHealth.org [Internet]*. Institute for Quality and Efficiency in Health Care (IQWiG). https://www.ncbi.nlm.nih.gov/books/NBK543221/

36. Jaffray, D. A., & Gospodarowicz, M. K. (2015). Radiation Therapy for Cancer. In H. Gelband, P. Jha, R. Sankaranarayanan, & S. Horton (Eds.), *Cancer: Disease Control Priorities, Third Edition (Volume 3)*. The International Bank for Reconstruction and Development / The World Bank. http://www.ncbi.nlm.nih.gov/books/NBK343621/

37. Jiang, J., Srivastava, S., & Zhang, J. (2019). Starve Cancer Cells of Glutamine: Break the Spell or Make a Hungry Monster? *Cancers, 11*(6), 804. https://doi.org/10.3390/cancers11060804

38. Kahl, K. L. (2020). Nivolumab/Ipilimumab Combo Yields Durable Efficacy in Advanced NSCLC. *Oncology (Williston Park, N.Y.), 34*(7), 254.

39. Kassovska-Bratinova, S., Fukao, T., Song, X. Q., Duncan, A. M., Chen, H. S., Robert, M. F., Pérez-Cerdá, C., Ugarte, M., Chartrand, C., Vobecky, S., Kondo, N., & Mitchell, G. A. (1996). Succinyl CoA: 3-oxoacid CoA transferase (SCOT): human cDNA cloning, human chromosomal mapping to 5p13, and mutation detection in a SCOT-deficient patient. *American Journal of Human Genetics, 59*(3), 519–528.

40. Kasznicki, J., Sliwinska, A., & Drzewoski, J. (2014). Metformin in cancer prevention and therapy. *Annals of Translational Medicine, 2*(6), 57.

https://doi.org/10.3978/j.issn.2305-5839.2014.06.01

41. Keenan, M., & Chi, J.-T. (2015). Alternative Fuels for Cancer Cells. *Cancer Journal (Sudbury, Mass.)*, *21*(2), 49–55. https://doi.org/10.1097/PPO.0000000000000104

42. Koo, M. M., Swann, R., McPhail, S., Abel, G. A., Elliss-Brookes, L., Rubin, G. P., & Lyratzopoulos, G. (2020). Presenting symptoms of cancer and stage at diagnosis: Evidence from a cross-sectional, population-based study. *The Lancet. Oncology*, *21*(1), 73–79. https://doi.org/10.1016/S1470-2045(19)30595-9

43. Kurbacher, C. M., Wagner, U., Kolster, B., Andreotti, P. E., Krebs, D., & Bruckner, H. W. (1996). Ascorbic acid (vitamin C) improves the antineoplastic activity of doxorubicin, cisplatin, and paclitaxel in human breast carcinoma cells in vitro. *Cancer Letters*, *103*(2), 183–189. https://doi.org/10.1016/0304-3835(96)04212-7

44. Li, Y.-Q., Zheng, Z., Liu, Q.-X., Lu, X., Zhou, D., Zhang, J., Zheng, H., & Dai, J.-G. (2021). Repositioning of Antiparasitic Drugs for Tumor Treatment. *Frontiers in Oncology*, *11*, 670804. https://doi.org/10.3389/fonc.2021.670804

45. Liberti, M. V., & Locasale, J. W. (2016). The Warburg Effect: How Does it Benefit Cancer Cells? *Trends in Biochemical Sciences*, *41*(3), 211–218. https://doi.org/10.1016/j.tibs.2015.12.001

46. Liu, Y., & Zeng, G. (2012). Cancer and Innate Immune System Interactions: Translational Potentials for Cancer Immunotherapy. *Journal of Immunotherapy (Hagerstown, Md. : 1997)*, *35*(4), 299–308. https://doi.org/10.1097/CJI.0b013e3182518e83

47. Lundström-Stadelmann, B., Rufener, R., & Hemphill, A. (2020). Drug repurposing applied: Activity of the anti-malarial mefloquine against Echinococcus multilocularis. *International Journal for Parasitology: Drugs and Drug Resistance*, *13*, 121–129. https://doi.org/10.1016/j.ijpddr.2020.06.002

48. Ma, M., & Baumgartner, M. (2014). Intracellular Theileria annulata Promote Invasive

Cell Motility through Kinase Regulation of the Host Actin Cytoskeleton. *PLoS Pathogens*, *10*(3), e1004003. https://doi.org/10.1371/journal.ppat.1004003

49. Marin, J. J. G., Romero, M. R., Blazquez, A. G., Herraez, E., Keck, E., & Briz, O. (2009). Importance and limitations of chemotherapy among the available treatments for gastrointestinal tumours. *Anti-Cancer Agents in Medicinal Chemistry*, *9*(2), 162–184. https://doi.org/10.2174/187152009787313828

50. McDaniel, S. H., Morse, D. S., Edwardsen, E. A., Taupin, A., Gurnsey, M. G., Griggs, J. J., Shields, C. G., & Reis, S. (2021). Empathy and boundary turbulence in cancer communication. *Patient Education and Counseling*, *104*(12), 2944–2951. https://doi.org/10.1016/j.pec.2021.04.002

51. Medina-Lara, A., Grigore, B., Lewis, R., Peters, J., Price, S., Landa, P., Robinson, S., Neal, R., Hamilton, W., & Spencer, A. E. (2020). Cancer diagnostic tools to aid decision-making in primary care: Mixed-methods systematic reviews and cost-effectiveness analysis. *Health Technology Assessment (Winchester, England)*, *24*(66), 1–332. https://doi.org/10.3310/hta24660

52. Melenotte, C., Epelboin, L., Million, M., Hubert, S., Monsec, T., Djossou, F., Mège, J.-L., Habib, G., & Raoult, D. (2019). Acute Q Fever Endocarditis: A Paradigm Shift Following the Systematic Use of Transthoracic Echocardiography During Acute Q Fever. *Clinical Infectious Diseases: An Official Publication of the Infectious Diseases Society of America*, *69*(11), 1987–1995. https://doi.org/10.1093/cid/ciz120

53. Mussa, A., Mohd Idris, R. A., Ahmed, N., Ahmad, S., Murtadha, A. H., Tengku Din, T. A. D. A. A., Yean, C. Y., Wan Abdul Rahman, W. F., Mat Lazim, N., Uskoković, V., Hajissa, K., Mokhtar, N. F., Mohamud, R., & Hassan, R. (2022). High-Dose Vitamin C for Cancer Therapy. *Pharmaceuticals*, *15*(6), 711. https://doi.org/10.3390/ph15060711

54. Park, D., Lee, J.-H., & Yoon, S.-P. (2022). Anti-cancer effects of fenbendazole on 5-fluorouracil-resistant colorectal cancer cells. *The Korean Journal of Physiology &*

Pharmacology : Official Journal of the Korean Physiological Society and the Korean Society of Pharmacology, *26*(5), 377–387. https://doi.org/10.4196/kjpp.2022.26.5.377

55. Pawlowska, E., Szczepanska, J., & Blasiak, J. (2019). Pro- and Antioxidant Effects of Vitamin C in Cancer in correspondence to Its Dietary and Pharmacological Concentrations. *Oxidative Medicine and Cellular Longevity*, *2019*, 7286737. https://doi.org/10.1155/2019/7286737

56. Peng, F., Wang, J.-H., Fan, W.-J., Meng, Y.-T., Li, M.-M., Li, T.-T., Cui, B., Wang, H.-F., Zhao, Y., An, F., Guo, T., Liu, X.-F., Zhang, L., Lv, L., Lv, D.-K., Xu, L.-Z., Xie, J.-J., Lin, W.-X., Lam, E. W.-F., … Liu, Q. (2018). Glycolysis gatekeeper PDK1 reprograms breast cancer stem cells under hypoxia. *Oncogene*, *37*(8), 1062–1074. https://doi.org/10.1038/onc.2017.368

57. Peng, Y., Wang, Y., Zhou, C., Mei, W., & Zeng, C. (2022). PI3K/Akt/mTOR Pathway and Its Role in Cancer Therapeutics: Are We Making Headway? *Frontiers in Oncology*, *12*, 819128. https://doi.org/10.3389/fonc.2022.819128

58. Pittman, R. N. (2011). Oxygen Transport. In *Regulation of Tissue Oxygenation*. Morgan & Claypool Life Sciences. https://www.ncbi.nlm.nih.gov/books/NBK54103/

59. Rajarajeswaran, P., & Vishnupriya, R. (2009). Exercise in cancer. *Indian Journal of Medical and Paediatric Oncology : Official Journal of Indian Society of Medical & Paediatric Oncology*, *30*(2), 61–70. https://doi.org/10.4103/0971-5851.60050

60. Rezaei Zonooz, S., Hasani, M., Morvaridzadeh, M., Beatriz Pizarro, A., Heydari, H., Yosaee, S., Rezamand, G., & Heshmati, J. (2021). Effect of alpha-lipoic acid on oxidative stress parameters: A systematic review and meta-analysis. *Journal of Functional Foods*, *87*, 104774. https://doi.org/10.1016/j.jff.2021.104774

61. Saini, R. (2011). Coenzyme Q10: The essential nutrient. *Journal of Pharmacy and Bioallied Sciences*, *3*(3), 466–467. https://doi.org/10.4103/0975-7406.84471

62. Sawant, M., Baydoun, M., Creusy, C., Chabé, M., Viscogliosi, E., Certad, G., &

Benamrouz-Vanneste, S. (2020). Cryptosporidium and Colon Cancer: Cause or Consequence? *Microorganisms*, *8*(11), 1665. https://doi.org/10.3390/microorganisms8111665

63. Schöllkopf, C., Melbye, M., Munksgaard, L., Smedby, K. E., Rostgaard, K., Glimelius, B., Chang, E. T., Roos, G., Hansen, M., Adami, H.-O., & Hjalgrim, H. (2008). Borrelia infection and risk of non-Hodgkin lymphoma. *Blood*, *111*(12), 5524–5529. https://doi.org/10.1182/blood-2007-08-109611

64. Seltzer, E. S., Watters, A. K., MacKenzie, D., Granat, L. M., & Zhang, D. (2020). Cannabidiol (CBD) as a Promising Anti-Cancer Drug. *Cancers*, *12*(11), 3203. https://doi.org/10.3390/cancers12113203

65. Semeniuk, G., Bahadini, B., Ahn, E., Zain, J., Cheng, J., Govindarajan, A., Rose, J., & Lee, R. T. (2023). Integrative Oncology and the Clinical Care Network: Challenges and Opportunities. *Journal of Clinical Medicine*, *12*(12), 3946. https://doi.org/10.3390/jcm12123946

66. Seyfried, T. N., Flores, R. E., Poff, A. M., & D'Agostino, D. P. (2014). Cancer as a metabolic disease: Implications for novel therapeutics. *Carcinogenesis*, *35*(3), 515–527. https://doi.org/10.1093/carcin/bgt480

67. Seyfried, T. N., & Shelton, L. M. (2010). Cancer as a metabolic disease. *Nutrition & Metabolism*, *7*, 7. https://doi.org/10.1186/1743-7075-7-7

68. Shin, M. S., Park, H.-J., Maeda, T., Nishioka, H., Fujii, H., & Kang, I. (2019). The Effects of AHCC®, a Standardized Extract of Cultured Lentinura edodes Mycelia, on Natural Killer and T Cells in Health and Disease: Reviews on Human and Animal Studies. *Journal of Immunology Research*, *2019*, 3758576. https://doi.org/10.1155/2019/3758576

69. Shishodia, S., Amin, H. M., Lai, R., & Aggarwal, B. B. (2005). Curcumin (diferuloylmethane) inhibits constitutive NF-kappaB activation, induces G1/S arrest,

suppresses proliferation, and induces apoptosis in mantle cell lymphoma. *Biochemical*

Pharmacology, 70(5), 700–713. https://doi.org/10.1016/j.bcp.2005.04.043

70. Shuel, S. L. (2022). Targeted cancer therapies. *Canadian Family Physician, 68*(7), 515–518. https://doi.org/10.46747/cfp.6807515

71. Singh, A. K., Singh, S. K., Nandi, M. K., Mishra, G., Maurya, A., Rai, A., Rai, G. K., Awasthi, R., Sharma, B., & Kulkarni, G. T. (2019). Berberine: A Plant-derived Alkaloid with Therapeutic Potential to Combat Alzheimer's disease. *Central Nervous System Agents in Medicinal Chemistry, 19*(3), 154–170. https://doi.org/10.2174/1871524919666190820160053

72. Song, B., Kim, K. J., & Ki, S. H. (2022). Experience with and perceptions of non-prescription anthelmintics for cancer treatments among cancer patients in South Korea: A cross-sectional survey. *PLoS ONE, 17*(10), e0275620. https://doi.org/10.1371/journal.pone.0275620

73. Sordo-Bahamonde, C., Lorenzo-Herrero, S., Gonzalez-Rodriguez, A. P., Martínez-Pérez, A., Rodrigo, J. P., García-Pedrero, J. M., & Gonzalez, S. (2023). Chemo-Immunotherapy: A New Trend in Cancer Treatment. *Cancers, 15*(11). https://doi.org/10.3390/cancers15112912

74. Spinelli, J. B., & Haigis, M. C. (2018). The Multifaceted Contributions of Mitochondria to Cellular Metabolism. *Nature Cell Biology, 20*(7), 745–754. https://doi.org/10.1038/s41556-018-0124-1

75. Suissa, S., & Azoulay, L. (2012). Metformin and the Risk of Cancer. *Diabetes Care, 35*(12), 2665–2673. https://doi.org/10.2337/dc12-0788

76. Sung, B., Chung, H. Y., & Kim, N. D. (2016). Role of Apigenin in Cancer Prevention via the Induction of Apoptosis and Autophagy. *Journal of Cancer Prevention, 21*(4), 216–226. https://doi.org/10.15430/JCP.2016.21.4.216

77. Sung, J. J. Y., Ho, J. M. W., Chan, F. C. H., & Tsoi, K. K. F. (2019). Low-dose aspirin

can reduce colorectal cancer mortality after surgery: A 10-year follow-up of 13 528 colorectal cancer patients. *Journal of Gastroenterology and Hepatology*, *34*(6), 1027–1034. https://doi.org/10.1111/jgh.14562

78. Tan-Shalaby, J. (2017). Ketogenic Diets and Cancer: Emerging Evidence. *Federal Practitioner*, *34*(Suppl 1), 37S-42S.

79. Teoli, D., Schoo, C., & Kalish, V. B. (2023). Palliative Care. In *StatPearls*. StatPearls Publishing. http://www.ncbi.nlm.nih.gov/books/NBK537113/

80. Tewari, D., Majumdar, D., Vallabhaneni, S., & Bera, A. K. (2017). Aspirin induces cell death by directly modulating mitochondrial voltage-dependent anion channel (VDAC). *Scientific Reports*, *7*, 45184. https://doi.org/10.1038/srep45184

81. Thanee, M., Padthaisong, S., Suksawat, M., Dokduang, H., Phetcharaburanin, J., Klanrit, P., Titapun, A., Namwat, N., Wangwiwatsin, A., Sa-ngiamwibool, P., Khuntikeo, N., Saya, H., & Loilome, W. (2021). Sulfasalazine modifies metabolic profiles and enhances cisplatin chemosensitivity on cholangiocarcinoma cells in in vitro and in vivo models. *Cancer & Metabolism*, *9*(1), 11. https://doi.org/10.1186/s40170-021-00249-6

82. Wargo, J. A., Reuben, A., Cooper, Z. A., Oh, K. S., & Sullivan, R. J. (2015). Immune Effects of Chemotherapy, Radiation, and Targeted Therapy and Opportunities for Combination With Immunotherapy. *Seminars in Oncology*, *42*(4), 601–616. https://doi.org/10.1053/j.seminoncol.2015.05.007

83. Welch, D. R., & Hurst, D. R. (2019). Defining the Hallmarks of Metastasis. *Cancer Research*, *79*(12), 3011–3027. https://doi.org/10.1158/0008-5472.CAN-19-0458

84. Welton, S., Minty, R., O'Driscoll, T., Willms, H., Poirier, D., Madden, S., & Kelly, L. (2020). Intermittent fasting and weight loss. *Canadian Family Physician*, *66*(2), 117–125.

85. Xu, D., Hu, M.-J., Wang, Y.-Q., & Cui, Y.-L. (2019). Antioxidant Activities of

Quercetin and Its Complexes for Medicinal Application. *Molecules, 24*(6), 1123. https://doi.org/10.3390/molecules24061123

86. Zhou, Y., Li, X., Luo, W., Zhu, J., Zhao, J., Wang, M., Sang, L., Chang, B., & Wang, B. (2022). Allicin in Digestive System Cancer: From Biological Effects to Clinical Treatment. *Frontiers in Pharmacology, 13,* 903259. https://doi.org/10.3389/fphar.2022.903259

****

Made in the USA
Las Vegas, NV
21 December 2024

35fd993f-6bb5-4cc2-864b-13c671d8bc3dR02